P9-CEU-716

Jewish Values
in Bioethics

Jewish Values in Bioethics

Edited by

Rabbi Levi Meier, Ph.D.

Cedars-Sinai Medical Center
Los Angeles, California

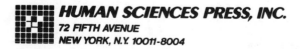 **HUMAN SCIENCES PRESS, INC.**
72 FIFTH AVENUE
NEW YORK, N.Y. 10011-8004

Dedicated
to the Memory
of
Max Martin Salick

Copyright © 1986 by Human Sciences Press, Inc.
72 Fifth Avenue, New York, New York 10011

All rights reserved. No part of this work may be reproduced or utilized in
any form or by any means, electronic or mechanical, including
photocopying, microfilm and recording, or by any information storage
and retrieval system without permission in writing from the publisher.

Printed in the United States of America
987654321

Library of Congress Cataloging-in-Publication Data

Jewish values in bioethics.

  Bibliography: p. 190
  Includes Index.
  1. Medical ethics. 2. Ethics, Jewish. 3. Bioethics.
4. Medicine—Religious aspects—Judaism. I. Meier, Levi.
R725.57.J49   1986   296.3'85   86-11395
ISBN 0-89885-299-4

Contents

W
50
J 595
1986

3 0001 00167 9283   16830487

PART II

Contributors

RABBI J. DAVID BLEICH, Ph.D.
Professor of Talmud
Yeshiva University, New York
Professor of Law
Benjamin Cardozo School of Law, New York

RABBI DAVID M. FELDMAN, D.H.L.
Chairman
Committee on Medical Ethics
Federation of Jewish Philanthropies, New York

VIKTOR E. FRANKL, M.D., Ph.D.
Founder of Logotherapy
The Third Viennese School of Psychotherapy
Vienna, Austria

RABBI IRVING GREENBERG, Ph.D.
President
National Jewish Resource Center, New York

SIR IMMANUEL JAKOBOVITS, Ph.D.
Chief Rabbi
The British Commonwealth of Nations

RABBI LEVI MEIER, Ph.D.
Chaplain
Cedars-Sinai Medical Center
Los Angeles, California
Psychotherapist in private practice

RABBI EMANUEL RACKMAN, Ph.D.
President
Bar-Ilan University, Israel

FRED ROSNER, M.D.
Director
Department of Medicine
Queen's Hospital Center, New York

Professor of Medicine
State University of New York at Stony Brook

ELIE WIESEL
Andrew Mellon Professor in the Humanities
Boston University

Chairman
United States Holocaust Memorial Council

About the Max Martin Salick Lectureship

The Max Martin Salick Lectures in Medical Ethics are a regular part of the academic program at Cedars-Sinai Medical Center in Los Angeles. They are dedicated to the memory of the husband of Blanche, the father of Allen, Bernard, and Reneé, and the grandfather of Ian, Adrienne, Nicholas, Gabriella, Elizabeth, and Anna-Martine. He died at the Medical Center at age seventy-two, after a brief but devastating battle with cancer.

Although he was born in the United States, he was sent to the "Old World" yeshivas in Hungary-Rumania for his schooling; and thus had little formal secular education. He established himself as a young adult in New York's Lower East Side, and after making and losing a fortune in the Depression, he returned to Europe to visit his family. There he met his future wife, Blanche, and shortly after their wedding, returned to the United States to earn the money for her to join him. The young couple were reunited in the United States and raised a family.

Max Martin Salick was a family man in the old tradition, with few interests apart from wife, children, grandchildren, and Judaism. Throughout a life devoted to reading, he became well-versed in philosophy, literature, and history. He loved to engage family and friends in discussions of Jewish ethics and history, and how it related to modern day life.

When he became ill, he remained cheerful, courageous, and optimistic to the end. He spoke of returning to work, even when he must have known that he never would. It is to the memory of this self-educated man, devoted husband, father, and grandfather, that we lovingly dedicate these lectures.

The Salick Family

Permissions

Gratitude is hereby expressed to the following for granting permission to reprint copyrighted materials:

"Code and No-Code: A Psychological Analysis and the Viewpoint of Jewish Law," by Levi Meier. From *Legal and Ethical Aspects of Treating Critically and Terminally Ill Patients*. Edited by A. Edward Doudera and J. Douglas Peters. Published in cooperation with the American Society of Law and Medicine, Association of University Programs in Health Administration and Health Administration Press, the University of Michigan, 1982.

"Filial Responsibility to the Senile Parent: A Jewish Approach," by Levi Meier. From *Journal of Psychology and Judaism,* Fall, 1977, 2(1), pp. 45–53. Copyright 1977 by Levi Meier. Reprinted by permission of Levi Meier. Reprinted from *Spiritual Well-Being of the Elderly*. Edited by James A. Thorson and Thomas C. Cook, Jr., 1977. Courtesy of Charles C. Thomas, Publisher, Springfield, Illinois. Reprinted from *A Psychology-Judaism Reader*. Edited by Reuven P. Bulka and Moshe HaLevi Spero, 1982. Courtesy of Charles C. Thomas, Publisher, Springfield, Illinois.

Man's Search For Meaning (Revised and updated), pp. 170–176. Copyright 1984 by Viktor Frankl. Reprinted by permission of Beacon Press, Boston, Massachusetts.

"Visiting the Sick: An Authentic Encounter," by Levi Meier. From *Bulletin of the American Protestant Hospital Association*. Special Edition on Pastoral Care. Proceedings of the Annual Convention, College of Chaplains. Edited by Charles D. Phillips. Volume XLIII, Number 2. Anaheim, California, 1979.

Acknowledgements

Numerous people have assisted me in the task of compiling and editing this book. First and foremost is Lewis Van Gelder, who in his meticulous and methodological way, has critically read and improved on the various authors' style.

The family of Max Martin Salick to whom this book is dedicated, has generously supported the special lectureships on Jewish medical ethics.

The staff of the word processing center and my secretary, Josie Bonorris.

To the Board of Rabbis of Southern California and to Jewish Federation Council of Greater Los Angeles for cooperating in our mutual endeavors.

The administration and Board of Directors of Cedars-Sinai Medical Center for constantly encouraging and facilitating my work as chaplain.

To Steve Broidy, founding life Chairman of Cedars-Sinai Medical Center, Robert L. Spencer, Chairman of the Cedars-Sinai Board of Directors, Stuart J. Marylander, President of Cedars-Sinai, and Larry Baum, Vice President for Community Relations of Cedars-Sinai Medical Center, who with their vision have not only cooperated but have also participated in the spiritual well-being of the patients of the Medical Center with professionalism and dedication.

The patients, physicians, and nurses who have frequently approached me with their very difficult questions and complex situations.

To my revered teacher and mentor, Rabbi Joseph B. Soloveitchik, who through his struggle in integrating Western civilization and Judaism has served as an inspiration and guide to all of his disciples.

To Ms. Norma Fox, editor-in-chief of Human Sciences Press, and her staff for sharing their knowledge, experience, and expertise in an amicable manner.

To my mother-in-law, Mrs. Belle Yarmish, who graciously opened her home to the distinguished lecturers in the medical ethics conferences.

To my brother, Rabbi Menachem Meier, Ph.D., with whom I have discussed many aspects of Jewish law. To my brother-in-law, Robert E. Levine, M.D., with whom I have discussed many aspects of medical ethics.

To my father, Alfred Meier, of blessed memory, and to my mother, Frieda Meier, who has always given me encouragement and fortitude.

To my dear wife, Marcie, and our four children—Chana, Yosef Asher, Malka Mindel, and Yitzchak Shlomo—who have added excitement, joy, and love to my life.

Preface

I am proud to present the following collection of contributions, based on the Max Martin Salick memorial lectureship on Jewish medical ethics, which indicate the *infinite* value of life and, it is hoped, will convey the style and atmosphere of the lectures.

In chapter 1 I discuss the dimension of meaning which death confers upon life.

Chapter 2 describes the circumstances under which a patient is to be resuscitated after he has suffered a cardiac or respiratory arrest.

Dr. Fred Rosner (chapter 3) and Rabbi David Bleich (chapter 4) discuss the issues involved in experimental treatment.

Chapter 5 deals with the responsibility of adult children to their aged parents in the unfortunate situation in which the parent is chronically senile.

In chapter 6 Sir Immanuel Jakobovits, the pioneer in the field of Jewish medical ethics, shares with us his views on "truth telling" and on the prolongation of life for the terminally ill patient.

Elie Wiesel, the foremost thinker on the Holocaust, discusses the special sensitivity which is required to care for a Holocaust survivor and his family in chapter 7.

In chapter 8, Dr. Viktor E. Frankl draws upon his personal and clinical experience to show how one can cope with suffering in a meaningful way.

Rabbi Irving Greenberg, in chapter 9, demonstrates the

special qualities that physicians must cultivate in order to practice medicine ethically. He emphasizes that through the practice of medicine, we perfect the world and become co-partners with God.

Rabbi Emanuel Rackman (chapter 10) discusses the process and methodology in Jewish law whereby medical ethical decisions are arrived at. He demonstrates that while the principles of Jewish law are unchanging, their application to specific situations may vary.

Rabbi David Feldman (chapter 11) shows how the principles of Jewish law can apply to contemporary innovations in reproductive techniques.

Finally, in chapter 12, I discuss the special sensitivity which is required when visiting the sick.

It is to be hoped that these twelve chapters will sensitize and guide the physician and patient alike in thinking through these most complex issues.

Rabbi Levi Meier, Ph.D.

Foreword

Traditionally, the physician has been a "student" of nature. Indeed, in ancient times faculties of medicine were representative not only of the natural sciences, but also of the physical and theoretical sciences, as well as of those disciplines now referred to as the biological sciences. Faculties of medicine were concerned with knowledge bearing on the relation of man to nature. Law and its extension to politics related man to man and society to society. Theology, expounding the relation of man and nature to God, addressed those actions of men that would appear to be ethically acceptable to a supreme power.

The title "doctor," generally used in the United States to denote practitioners of medicine, is commonly restricted to those of superior knowledge. In the deeper meaning of the term, the professional ideal incorporates knowledge, teaching, and service to their fellowmen. These ideals are formulated in the Hippocratic Oath, in which the commitment of the physician to his patient and his profession is strongly underscored. The relation of medical art and practice to nature characterized the writings of the ancient Greeks. The immense complexity of human biology and medicine was recognized, and the role of the physician was, and is, to place the patient in an optimal relation for natural healing. The admonition of Hippocrates "to do good and to do no harm" has been expanded, even in modern times, "to cure sometimes, to harm never, and to comfort always."

The physician, and perhaps more importantly, the true "doctor" is being called to participate in major decisions of great moral, ethical, and social magnitude. Further, physicians in practice have of necessity become participatory as individuals in these ethical questions. While biological sciences are both the source and the reflection of medical knowledge and research, they also are used to preserve the health of individuals. Hence medicine today is impaled upon societal issues outside of its unique responsibility to the individual. Birth control, abortion, life in the disabled newborn, definition of death, organ transplantation, life-support systems, and the coma patient—these are but some of the complex and unresolved ethical issues which confront the present-day physician.

In medicine, as in law, no general rule fits all cases. As a result, the "rights" of the individual, reflected by major issues of appropriate recovery for inflicted injury ("malpractice") confronts physicians daily. In many ways, a return to the principle of natural philosophy in which the general order of things (nature) "also takes care of men if they will have patience" may be desirable. But society will not agree to let nature take care of medical decision making; and medicine, together with law and theology, must combine their considerations to consider and attempt resolution of these complex and morally disturbing questions.

Traditional Jewish ethics and scholarship clearly stand in the forefront of moral thought. Here, societal and individual wants have been placed against fundamental principles of behavior. This series of Salick lectures, so ably presented by Rabbi Levi Meier, offer a sound base for decisions. Indeed, we are bound to use considered ethical principles derived from our past as evidence for our future. These principles so well presented on the important issues considered in this monograph can provide the physician guidance in the moral, ethical, and legal dilemmas which face him in the future.

H. J. C. Swan, M.D., Ph.D.
Professor of Medicine
University of California, Los Angeles
School of Medicine

Director of Cardiology
Cedars-Sinai Medical Center
Los Angeles, California

Part I

1

Introduction

Rabbi Levi Meier, Ph.D.

QUALITY OF LIFE

"Though the physicality of death destroys an individual, the *idea* of death can save him" (Yalom, 1980). An awareness of death moves one away from trivial preoccupations and concerns and provides life with depth and substance from an entirely different perspective.

An awareness of the importance of medical ethics allows physicians and their patients to focus on the most profound and pressing issues relating to the preservation of life. Though the issues of medical ethics may appear very complex, remote, and esoteric, their real-life application is a vital, everyday part of modern medical treatment. Indeed, both the quality and quantity of life are at the root of medical ethics.

Quantity of life is defined as the duration of one's existence. But what are the parameters and criteria of *quality* of life? In the realm of medical ethics, this is the *quintessential* area of investigation. Physicians, bioethicists, attorneys, and clergy have not ventured into this realm in a methodological manner. They have arrived at their conclusions from a subjective and personal stance. Frequently, the professionals have been guided by "situational ethics:" i.e., doing what appears appropriate in a particular situation under particular circumstances.

Nowhere are the ethical dilemmas involving the quality of life more pressing than with respect to death and dying. A terminal cancer patient who is experiencing great pain suffers cardiac arrest; should the patient be resuscitated? A family member with a life-threatening illness refuses to undergo treatment; should treatment be administered in violation of the patient's expressed wishes?

The triumphs of modern medicine are everywhere. Achievements such as open-heart surgery and organ transplants, dialysis machines that substitute for the kidneys, pacemakers that regulate the beating of the heart, and vaccines that have made once-dreaded diseases almost forgotten words have become commonplace. The new technologies do not always cure, but sometimes merely prolong the dying process. The irony of modern medicine is that with the new technologies that vastly expand the range of the possible has also come the anguish of deciding when it is appropriate to use those capabilities.

The Indignity of "Death with Dignity"

In trying to grapple with these most difficult issues, some ethicists have introduced phrases such as "death with dignity." These proponents have intentionally used a phrase that evokes compassion and empathy. Paul Ramsey (1974) accentuates the absurdity of the phrase by entitling his article *The Indignity of "Death with Dignity."* In contrast to the theme of "death with dignity" stands Dylan Thomas's

(1953) famous poem for his father, *Do Not Go Gentle Into That Good Night,* in which he urges, "Old age should burn and rage at the close of day;/Rage, Rage against the dying of the light."

"Death with dignity" is ultimately a contradiction in terms. Disease, injury, and congenital defects are—like death—a part of life. Yet there is no campaign for accepting those things with dignity. Nor is there emphasis on "suffering with dignity." All of these occurrences, including death, are enemies and violations of human nobility. Grief over death, as well as the biopsychosocial pain of dying, needs to be *acknowledged.*

Rabbi Soloveitchik's View on Death

The antithetical relationship of death to life is reflected in the thought of Rabbi Joseph Soloveitchik (1983). "We have stated that Judaism, as reflected in the *Halakhah,* has a negative attitude toward death. A person is obligated to rend his garment and mourn for his relative. The *Halakhah* has established certain units of time with regard to mourning: the first day (on which mourning, according to many *rishonim* [early medieval authorities], is a biblical commandment), 7 days, 30 days, 12 months. The *onen,* a mourner on the day of death, is forbidden to eat any sacred offerings; moreover, the mourner does not have any sacrifices offered up on his behalf during the entire 7-day mourning period. The high priest is forbidden to let his hair grow and rend his garment for his dead relative, for preoccupation with the memory of the dead desecrates the holiness of the Temple and of the high priesthood. Indeed, many *rishonim* exempted the high priest from all rites of mourning. Holiness is rooted and embedded in joy. "And ye shall rejoice before the Lord your God seven days" (Lev.

23:40), "and thou shalt rejoice in all the good" (Deut. 26:40), "and thou shalt be altogether joyful" (Deut, 16:15). Joy is the symbol of the real life in which the *Halakhah* is actualized. *Avelut,* mourning, and *aninut,* grief, however, are interwoven and bound up with the archopponent of holiness—death. Death and holiness constitute two contradictory verses, as it were, and the third harmonizing verse has yet to make its appearance. The Gaon of Vilna, R. Joseph Dov Soloveitchik, his son, R. Hayyim, his grandson, R. Moses, and R. Elijah Pruzna (Feinstein) never visited cemeteries and never prostrated themselves upon the graves of their ancestors. The memory of death would have distracted them from their intensive efforts to study the Torah.

It is only against this background that we can comprehend a peculiar feature in the character of many great Jewish scholars and *halakhic* giants: the fear of death. *Halakhic* man is afraid of death; the dread of dissolution often seizes hold of him. My uncle, R. Meir Berlin (Bar-Ilan), related the following incident to me. He and R. Hayyim of Brisk once happened to be staying in the same hotel in Libau on the shore of the Baltic. One fine clear morning he arose at sunrise and went out on the balcony to find R. Hayyim sitting there, his head between his hands, his glance fixed upon the rays of the rising sun, entirely absorbed in the esthetic experience of such a glorious cosmic spectacle and at the same time overwhelmed by melancholy and black despair.

R. Berlin took hold of R. Hayyim's shoulder and shook it. "Why are you so troubled and disturbed, my master and teacher? Is something in particular responsible for your distress?"

"Yes," replied R. Hayyim, "I am reflecting upon the end of every man—death."

Halakhic man enjoyed the splendor of sunrise in the east and the swelling sea in the west, but this very experience, which portrayed in miniature the beauty of the cosmos as a whole and the joy of sheer existence, precipitated for him the deepest depression. The beauty and splendor of the world, on the one hand, and on the other, the fate of man, who can enjoy this mysterious magnificence for only a brief, fleeting moment, touched the chords of his sensitive heart by the tragic irony of the juxtaposition: a great and resplendent world, and man, "few of days, and full of trouble" (Job 14:1). The fear of death is transformed here into a quiet anguish, a silent pain, and a tender and delicate sadness intensified by the precious embellishment of a profound and lofty esthetic experience. However, the individual who undergoes such an exalted experience is not one who longs for transcendence, and yearns to break out of the realm of the concrete; for why should such a person be disheartened and grieved on account of the beauty of this world, which is but a pale reflection of a hidden, supernal existence. The *halakhic* man, who gazed at the first rays of the sun and reflected upon the beauty of the world and the nothingness of man, in an ecstatic mood of joy intermixed with tragedy, is a this-worldly man, an individual given over to concrete reality, who communicates with his Creator, not beyond the bounds of finitude, not in a holy, transcendent realm enwrapped in mystery, but rather in the very midst of the world and the fullness thereof.

"I said: I shall not see the Lord, even the Lord in the land of the living. . .For the nether-world cannot praise Thee: death cannot celebrate Thee: they that go down into the pit cannot hope for Thy truth. The living, the living, he shall praise Thee, as I do this day; the Father to the children shall make known Thy truth" (Isa. 38:11-19), sang King Hezekiah, when he recovered from his illness. "I shall not die, but live, and declare the works of the Lord" (Ps. 118:17), pleaded David, king of Israel, before his Creator. And the echo of these hymns still resounds through the world of *halakhah* ((pp. 35-37).

SUFFERING

The proponents of "death with dignity" also invoke concern for ameliorating the suffering of the dying patient.

The nature of suffering is a highly complex issue involving the individual's subjective pain-threshold and the value/meaning that is attached to the suffering (Meier, 1981). Marcel (1950), a Christian Existentialist, stated that "life is not a problem to be solved but rather a challenge to be lived." Rabbi Soloveitchik (1983), also an Existentialist, stated that "against my will I was created and against my will I shall die, but through my will I shall live." These two highly eloquent and succinct statements reflect an alternative approach to a dying man's excruciating suffering.

It is not uncommon for suffering to occur not only during the course of a disease but also as a result of its treatment. A cancer patient may seek relief through chemotherapy and radiation treatment. Even when these treatments are successful, the success sometimes brings with it terrible side effects that some patients claim are equal to the disease itself. Medical science presumes the Cartesian dualism of mind and body. Yet suffering is experienced by persons. The understanding of the place of the *person* in human illness requires a rejection of the historical dualism of mind and body. As long as the mind-body dichotomy is accepted, suffering is either subjective, and therefore not truly "real"—not within medicine's domain—or identified exclusively with bodily pain (Cassell, 1982). This distortion is itself an additional source of suffering.

The personal meaning which is identified with an illness affects the suffering of the patient. Rabbi Meier (1981) differentiated between the suffering of a patient with a chronic illness and a terminally ill patient. "Phenomenologically and existentially, a patient with a chronic ailment perceives his future suffering in the present (van den Berg, 1972). Van den Berg explains man's relationship to time by theorizing that future and past are embodied in the present. "The past is within the present: What WAS is the *way* it is appearing NOW. The future: what comes, the *way* it is meeting us now." (p. 91) A patient with a chronic ailment experiences not only present suffering, but also future anticipated suffering embodied in the present moment.

In contrast, a patient who is terminal experiences subjective death now, but not "eternal suffering." This experience of finiteness may motivate the patient to grow as a person and/or to achieve closure with his family and others with whom he has significant relationships. Even if this experience of finiteness brings depression, the patient knows that this depression is also finite and of temporary duration.

Therefore, wherever possible, suffering should be avoided or eliminated through medical care. But suffering should not be terminated by either "death with dignity," or an "easy death" (euthanasia).

Viktor Frankl (1983) stated that the concept of death gives meaning to life. How can there be any meaning to life in the face of the fundamental transitoriness of existence? The idea of death does not eliminate the meaning of life, but — on the contrary — enhances the meaning of life. If life was infinite, then everything could be delayed ad infinitum. Only under the pressure of the transitoriness of existence is one required to act immediately. It is only the potentialities that are passing. Once a possibility has been actualized, it exists forever. The past contains not only past experiences but also the sufferings courageously lived through.

When reflecting on one's life, a person tends to dwell on his misgivings and fears, and forgets to look at the grandeur of the past. There is no need to pity an old man because life is behind him; on the contrary, one would have to envy him. While young men have only possibilities before them, old people have their realities, which have already been actualized.

Frankl stated (1983) that life is meaningful in an unconditional sense, even under the most miserable conditions. Just as there is an unconditional meaningfulness to life, there is also an unconditional value to man. This unconditional value, or dignity, does not depend on any "usefulness" in terms of societal, family, or individual functions. Real dignity, including that of old or chronically sick people, relies on the values with which they have lived and on the meanings they have deposited into their personal pasts. This dignity cannot be deleted. Those who do not ascribe this unconditional value to old people, handicapped people, and disoriented people would have justified Hilter's euthanasia program of eliminating psychotic people. It is only this unconditional value of every person that restrains us.

"D equals S minus M," is Dr. Frankl's equation. *D*espair is *s*uffering without *m*eaning. If a person is unable to remove the current suffering, then one is mandated to try to impose a meaning upon suffering. Nobody can *give* meaning; one has to *find* meaning. Each and every individual may arrive at his or her own meaning.

It has been said that if a doctor treats two cases in the same way, then he has mistreated at least one of them. Everyone must find his own uniqueness to his situation. Doctors cannot prescribe meaning to a patient suffering from meaninglessness. Doctors can describe the process of what is going on in an individual in a given situation. The only thing doctors can do is to study the lives of people who seem to have found their "answers" as against those who have not.

The discovery of meaning in a life situation can be arrived at by three principal avenues. First, by doing something of creative value. Secondly, by experiencing something beautiful—through valuable research, scientific work, or through love. The third avenue is the most courageous. One may still find meaning precisely when confronted with a hopeless situation that cannot be changed. It is in this type of situation that a helpless victim has his greatest opportunity. He has the capacity to turn a tragedy into a personal triumph and accomplishment.

Dr. Frankl (1983) shares a moving story exemplifying how life is always a time of unparalleled potential for personal and interpersonal growth. A few years after World War II, a doctor examined a Jewish woman who wore a bracelet made of baby teeth, mounted in gold. A beautiful bracelet, the doctor remarked. Yes, the woman answered; you see, this tooth here belongs to Miriam, this one to Esther, and this one to Samuel. She mentioned the names of her 8 daughters and 1 son by age, nine children; and all of them had been taken to the gas chambers. Shocked, the doctor asked, "How can you live with such a bracelet?" Quietly, the Jewish woman replied, "I'm now in charge of an orphanage in Israel."

A QUEST FOR MEANING

Whatever solution is suggested in the various ethical dilemmas which are presented, the approach must be in consonance with the basic meaning of life which the patient has developed. There have been various theistic and atheistic approaches to this most basic issue (Yalom, 1980).

A common theme exemplifying a Jewish attitude to medical crises and ethical dilemmas is *engagement* in value-oriented activities. Man is required to take a leap into commitment and action. Meaning must be pursued obliquely. A sense of meaningfulness is a by-product of engagement.

Wholehearted engagement enhances the possibility of

one's completing the patterning of the events of one's life in some coherent fashion.

The Talmud teaches how engagement in the last moment of a person's life can give meaning to suffering. "Rabbi Hanina ben Teradyon [a victim of second-century Roman persecution] was wrapped in the Torah from which he had been teaching and placed on a pyre of green brushwood, and his chest was drenched with water to prolong the agony. His disciples, watching the flames dancing over their beloved teacher, asked: 'Master, what do you see?' He replied: 'I see parchment burning, while the letters of the Torah soar upward.' His disciples then advised him to open his mouth that the fire might enter and the sooner put an end to his suffering; but he refused to do so, saying: 'It is best that He who has given life should also take it away; no one may hasten his own death.' The executioner removed the wet sponge and fanned the flame, thus accelerating the end, and then plunged himself into the fire" (Birnbaum, 1951).[1]

The narrative of the martyred sage exemplifies that any deliberate acceleration of the final release is prohibited. Rabbi Hanina ben Teradyon refused to follow his disciples' advice to open his mouth to the flames in order to speed his death. Jewish law emphasizes the mitigation of a patient's suffering, especially in the ordeal prior to death, *except at the cost of life itself*, for human life has infinite value (Jakobovits, 1975).

Rabbi Hanina's actions demonstrate that even one second before he became immortal, he achieved "temporal immortality" by having *engaged* in valued activities. Once again, he assumed his role as a teacher of Torah. This time it was not only by didactic methodology but also by example. He taught the quintessential lesson of Jewish medical ethics: life has *infinite* value. Even in the excruciating suffering of a terminally ill person, meaning can be found by engaging in immortal lessons for mankind. Through man's awareness of his finitude and precisely because of it, man can achieve "infinite immortality." Once he is deceased, man's life is not something of the distant past but of the everlasting example for future generations. Rabbi Hanina's teachings are immortal.

NOTE

1. "On their return, the Roman officials found Rabbi Hanina ben Teradyon sitting and occupying himself with the Torah, publicly gathering assemblies, and keeping the scroll of the Law in his bosom. Straightaway they took hold of him, wrapped him in the Scroll of the Law, placed bundles of branches round him and set them on fire. They then brought tufts of wool, which they soaked in water, and placed them over his heart, so that he should not expire quickly. His daughter exclaimed, "Father that I should see you in this state!" He replied, "If it were I alone being burnt it would have been a thing hard to bear; but now that I am burning together with the Scroll of the Law, He who will have regard for the plight of the Torah will also have regard for my plight." His disciples called out, "Rabbi, what do you see?' He answered them, "The parchments are being burnt but the letters are soaring on high." "Open then your mouth so that the fire may enter into you." He replied, "Let Him who gave my soul take it away, but no one should injure oneself." The executioner then said to him, "Rabbi, if I raise the flame and take away the tufts of wool from over your heart, will you cause me to enter into the life to come?" "Yes," he replied. "Then swear unto me!" He swore unto him. He thereupon raised the flame and removed the tufts of wool from over his heart, and his soul departed speedily. The executioner then jumped and threw himself into the fire. And a heavenly voice exclaimed: Rabbi Hanina ben Teradyon and the executioner have been assigned to the world to come (Babylonian Talmud, Abodah Zarah, 18A; original text of story).

REFERENCES

Babylonian Talmud, Abodah Zarah. London: The Soncino Press, 1935.

Birnbaum, P. *High holyday prayer book,* (P. Birnbaum, trans.): New York; Hebrew Publishing Company, 1951.

Cassell, E. J. The nature of suffering and the goals of medicine. *The New England Journal of Medicine,* 1982, *306,*(11), 639-645.

Frankl, V. E. *The meaning of suffering.* Videocassette, Health Science Information Center, Cedars-Sinai Medical Center, January 31, 1983.

Jakobovits, I. *Jewish medical ethics.* New York: Bloch Publishing Company, 1975.

Marcel, G. *The mystery of being.* Chicago: Regnery, 1950.

Meier, L. Chronic pain, suffering, and spirituality: The relationship between chronic pain, suffering, and different religious approaches. Unpublished dissertation, University of Southern California, 1981.

Ramsey, P. The indignity of "death with dignity." *Hasting Center Studies,* Vol. 2, No. 2, May 1974.

Soloveitchik, J. B. *Halakhic man.* (L. Kaplan, trans.), Philadelphia: The Jewish Publication Society of America, 1983. (First published in *Talpioth,* 1944, *1,* 651-735.)

Thomas, D. *The collected poems of Dylan Thomas.* New York: New Directions, 1953.

van den Berg, J H. *A different existence.* Pittsburgh: Duquesne University Press, 1972.

Yalom, I. D. *Existential psychotherapy.* New York: Basic Books, 1980.

2

Code and No-Code
A Psychological Analysis and the Viewpoint of Jewish Law

Rabbi Levi Meier, Ph.D.

The decision to write or not to write a no-code or DNR order for a patient is a complex issue. It involves the physician-patient relationship, the physician-family relationship, the rights of the patient and the moral choices of the physician. This paper will address the problem in terms of psychology and *halakha* (Jewish law).

Within the general context of the physician-patient relationship, it is understood that the patient's values, cultural background, and family orientation may differ from those of the physician. In areas where the patient's and physician's values differ dramatically, there is a range of possible modes of behavior. The physician can withdraw from the case, explaining that his or her value system cannot accommodate the patient's desires. The physician can attempt to impose his or her value system on the patient, overtly or subtly; or the physician can differentiate between personal values and professional behavior. Lawrence Kohlberg's analysis of moral development sheds light on the physician's dilemma in such cases (Kohlberg, 1958).

Kohlberg's theory distinguishes between the preconventional, conventional and postconventional stages of moral development. The preconventional stage is characterized by avoiding punishment and satisfying one's own needs. The conventional stage involves the acceptance of the values of the group. Frequently, one follows peer group standards, although group values also include those of the broader community, the state, or the nation. An act is right because it conforms with accepted laws. This is the law-and-order stage, which often leads to the position that national policy should be supported whether it is right or wrong. The postconventional stage goes beyond specific rules and extends to man's conscience. It is based on abstract ethical principles that are believed to have universal applicability.

Kohlberg's theory recognizes that individuals differ in their values and that a physician's behavior in treating a patient with values different from his or her own may involve:

1. withdrawing from the case because of a value conflict: this reflects the postconventional stage of moral development where a person's conscience dictates the choice;
2. imposing his or her view on the patient. This is not even an option, according to Kohlberg;
3. differentiating between his or her personal ethic and that of the patient, and accepting whatever the patient requests. This course of action reflects Kohlberg's conventional stage, whereby a physician accepts the values of the group. In this case, the group is represented by

every individual patient. This option would allow for a physician treating two patients with identical medical situations to write diametrically opposite orders, depending upon which patient requests a code and which patient requests a no-code. In informal and formal discussions, physicians, nurses, and other health professionals frequently justify this position by stating that medical care must be individualized. However, as significant as individualized medical care is, it appears that the moral reasoning in accepting the patient's different significant choices reflects the physician's acquiescence and delegation of this responsibility. Although this course of action is seemingly in accordance with Kohlberg's theory, it appears that in this situation, acquiescence to a patient's desire is not an ethical option.

What is the patient's right in determining his or her own status? Is every individual totally free, or not?

THE PATIENT'S RIGHT

The California Natural Death Act states,

> The Legislature finds that adult persons have the fundamental right to control the decisions relating to the rendering of their own medical care, including the decision to have life-sustaining procedures withheld or withdrawn in instances of terminal condition (*California Health and Safety Code* §7186).

Prima facie, it would appear that there should be no restraint imposed upon this right. In forensic psychiatry, however, there is precedent for the infringement of patients' rights. The Lanterman-Petris-Short Act of 1969 states that within a therapeutic relationship, confidentiality is necessary (*Cal-*

ifornia Welfare and Institutions Code § 5328). However, confidentiality may be violated in a variety of circumstances, such as when the therapist views the patient as suicidal, homicidal, and/or unable to take care of self (unable to provide shelter, food, clothing, etc.). In these cases, a therapist may inform the authorities of the mental state of the patient in order to commence commitment proceedings. The principle is that patients' rights are circumscribed when patients, because of their mental state, are not responsible for their decisions.

As chaplain of Cedars-Sinai Medical Center, I am currently seeing a terminal patient who has been diagnosed as having cancer of the colon and liver. She has requested a no-code and, for that matter, prefers no treatment at all to treatment that involves secondary pain and suffering. According to the Zung (1974) depression scale and the Beck (1974) depression scale, she appears to be severely depressed. Clinical interviews have substantiated these test results. She states that her life no longer has purpose and that she would like to die immediately. Shoud we ignore her psychological condition and accede to her wishes, or should we treat her?

I believe that the therapist-client relationship and the physician-patient relationship share many identical elements. Just as the therapist recognizes that a suicidal desire results from severe depression, a physician can understand that requests for no treatment may be highly motivated by depression. An otherwise healthy person can feel as depressed as a patient who has terminal cancer. We need to devise a method of decision making that takes this sort of problem into account. The principle behind the Lanterman-Petris-Short Act should be operative in other areas of medicine.

In theological terms, too, man's liberty is circumscribed.

Life is a gift which has been bestowed and only the One who bestowed it may take it back. It is true that life may involve a tremendous amount of pain and suffering, yet Gabriel Marcel (1950), a French existentialist, said that life is not a problem to be solved but rather a challenge to be lived. Viktor Frankl (1962), the founder of Logotherapy, claims that man must find meaning in his tragedy.

PHYSICIAN-PATIENT RELATIONSHIP

Sometimes a physician may say, "If this were my father, I would. . . ." Obviously, this statement comes from a very caring position, but it involves numerous problems. The most important of these is that the patient is not the physician's father. Also, there is frequently a discrepancy between what people say they will do and what they in fact do. Intentions are often modified when it is actually time to make decisions.

In a regular therapeutic situation, no therapist would tell a couple, "Yes, a divorce would be appropriate," or "No, you should stay together." No therapist would ever want such enormous power over a patient. Yet in a physician-patient relationship, which takes the form of a therapeutic alliance, the physician is at times very directive in issues that involve ethics.

PHYSICIAN-FAMILY RELATIONSHIP

A physician deals not only with a patient, but also with the family of the patient and the relationship of the patient to his or her family. When a major decision needs to be made and the patient is unable to communicate, the family's contribution is especially significant. Sometimes a family member of a terminally ill patient may respond in these ways:

1. "There is too much suffering and pain going on. Knowing the patient for the past 70 years, I can tell you that he has faced too much agony."
2. "The family is having a nervous breakdown. Not only is the patient going to die, but her relatives are in mental anguish."
3. "The patient is not functioning. This is not the Dad I knew. He is a different person. There will be no meaning for him in life in any case."

My response to these and similar situations is to differentiate between the patient's expressed need and the family's need. The family, quite understandably, feels completely helpless, which can lead to bitter frustration, anger, and resentment. This family is in need of mental health assistance, but their pressing need should not lead to a no-code order. My clinical experience has shown me that a few years after the patient has died, the family begins to ponder the sequence of events again in its entirety. Conflicts that frequently arise are expressed by such statements as:

1. "I should have gone to a different physician or at least had a second consultation."
2. "Perhaps with a different hospital and a better nursing staff, the situation would have been altered."
3. "Why didn't I have them take more medically aggressive action?" (Lo & Jonsen, 1980).

It is human nature to have some guilt feelings about past relationships. Perhaps these feelings can be modified if the physician concentrates primarily upon the patient's needs and provides mental health assistance for the patient's family.

THE JUDAIC TRADITION

Within Judaic tradition, life has infinite value—even a diminished life. The value of a human life is not based upon its potential usefulness to others or upon one's own well-being. It is an absolute value, even when life is accompanied by pain, suffering, and mental anguish.

Humans do not possess absolute titles to life. Each is responsible for preserving his/her own life and is obliged to seek food and sustenance to that end. When one is sick, he/she is similarly obliged to seek medical attention. People are never called upon to determine whether their lives are worth living. This Judaic tradition is in direct contrast to the 1979 *Report of the Committee on Policy for Do Not Resuscitate Decisions,* of Yale University School of Medicine, which classifies three approaches to the management of the terminally ill:

1. patients are to receive all curative and functional maintenance therapies as indicated and the primary goal is to achieve arrest, remission, or cure of the basic disease process;
2. if any curative therapy is in progress, it will be continued until its outcome has been determined, and further, no new therapy will be implemented. A DNR order is optional;
3. the goals of therapy are to comfort the patient as he is dying, and so a DNR order is appropriate.

In Jewish thought, the quality of the life to be preserved is never a factor to be taken into consideration. Neither is the survivor's life expectancy a controlling factor, nor is the patient's age. A ninety-three-year-old patient with terminal cancer receives the same management as a thirty-nine-year-old patient with terminal cancer. Thus, classifications 2 and 3 of the Yale Report are antithetical to Jewish law.

EXPERIMENTAL THERAPY AND HAZARDOUS
PROCEDURES

There is no basis in Judaism for a distinction between ordinary and extraordinary forms of therapy (Bleich, 1979). However, a distinction must be made between therapeutic procedures of proven efficacy and those of unproven therapeutic value. If a therapeutic procedure is of proven efficacy, then it is a moral and *halakhic* imperative. Man may no more abstain from the use of drugs to cure illness than he may abstain from food or drink. However, if the proposed therapy is of unproven value, then the patient may legitimately refuse treatment. This is true not only when the treatment itself is potentially hazardous, but also if there is reason to suspect that the proposed treatment may be harmful in any way. In such instances, treatment is discretionary.

Physicians may withhold otherwise mandatory treatment only when the patient has reached the state of *gesisah,* i.e., the patient has become moribund and death is imminent. Even at this stage, the patient (or *goses*) is regarded as a living person in every respect. One must not pry his jaws, anoint him, wash him, plug his orifices, remove the pillow from underneath him or place him on the ground (Shulhan Arukh, Yoreh De'ah 339:1).

THE MORIBUND PATIENT

Although euthanasia in any form is forbidden and the hastening of death, even by a matter of moments, is regarded as tantamount to murder, there is one situation in which treatment may be withheld from the moribund patient in order to provide for an unimpeded death. While the death of a *goses* may not be speeded, there is no obligation to perform any action which will lengthen the life of the patient in this state. This distinction between an active and passive act applies only to a *goses*. When a patient is in the death process, there is no obligation to heal. Therefore, Rabbi Moses Isserles permits the removal of anything which constitutes a hindrance to the departure of the soul (such as a clattering noise or salt upon his tongue), since such acts involve no active hastening of death, but only the removal of an impediment (Shulhan Arukh, Yoreh De'ah 339:1).

It cannot be overemphasized that even acts of omission are permitted only when the patient is in a state of *gesisah*. This leads one to ask how the *gesisah* can be differentiated from other states?

1. If the condition is reversible, there is an obligation to heal. When the moribund condition is irreversible, there is no obligation to continue treatment.
2. Any patient who may reasonably be deemed capable of potential survival for a period of 72 hours cannot be considered a *goses* (Shulhan Arukh, Yoreh De'ah 339:2).

It appears that this state is not determined by a patient's ability to survive solely by natural means for this period, unaided by drugs or mechanical equipment. The implication is that a *goses* is one who cannot, by any means, be maintained alive for a period of 72 hours. The conclusion is that, if it is medically possible to prolong life, the patient is indeed not a *goses*.

The Judaic Tradition and Contemporary Society

This paper argues for aggressive treatment of terminally ill patients, regardless of the extent of the impairment or the quality of life which may be preserved by such treatment. The Judaic tradition is well aware that the motivation of contemporary society, in seeking not to prolong life in some cases, is brotherly compassion and feelings of love and concern. Nevertheless, euthanasia, even if designed to put an end to unbearable suffering, is classified as murder. Despite the noble intent which prompts such an action, mercy killing is considered an unwarranted intervention in an area which must be governed only by God.

REFERENCES

Beck, A., Beamesdorfer, A. Assessment of depression: The depression inventory. In P. Pichot (Ed.), *Psychological measurement in psychopharmacology*. New York: Karger, 1974.

Bleich, J.D. The obligation to heal in the Judaic tradition: A comparative analysis. In F. Rosner & J.D. Bleich (Eds.), *Jewish bioethics*. New York: Sanhedrin Press, Hebrew Publishing Company, 1979.

California Health and Safety Code § 7186 (West Supp., St. Paul, Minnesota, 1985).

California Welfare and Institutions Code § 5328 (West, St. Paul, Minnesota, 1984).

Frankl, V. *Man's search for meaning: An introduction to logotherapy*. Boston: Beacon Press, 1962.

Kohlberg, L. The development of modes of moral thinking and choice in years ten to sixteen. Unpublished doctoral dissertation, University of Chicago, 1958.

Lo, B. & Jonsen, A.R. Ethical decisions in the care of a patient terminally ill with metastic cancer. January 1980. *Annals of Internal Medicine,92*(1), 107-111. (Wife of deceased man asked several months after his death whether she should have requested more aggressive treatment.)

Marcel, G. *The mystery of being*. Chicago: Regnery, 1950.

Report of the committee on policy for do not resuscitate decisions. R.J. Levine, M.D., Chairman. New Haven: Yale University school of Medicine, March 1979.

Shulhan Arukh, Yoreh De'ah 339:1

Shulhan Arukh, Yoreh De'ah 339:2

Zung, W.W.K. The measurements of affects: Depression and anxiety. In P. Pichot (Ed.), *Psychological measurement in psychopharmacology.* New York: Karger, 1974.

3

Risks versus Benefits in Treating the Gravely Ill Patient
Ethical and Religious Considerations

Fred Rosner, M.D.

*I*n Jewish tradition, a physician is given specific divine license to practice medicine. According to Maimonides and other codifiers of Jewish law, it is in fact obligatory for the physician to use his medical skills to heal the sick. Not only is the *physician* permitted and even obligated to minister to the sick, but the *patient* is also obligated to care for his own health and life. Man does not have title over his life or body. He is charged with preserving, dignifying, and hallowing that life. He must eat and drink to sustain himself; he must seek healing when he is ill.

Another cardinal principle in Judaism is that human life is of infinite value. The preservation of human life takes precedence over all biblical injunctions, with three exceptions: the prohibition of idolatry, murder, and incest. Life's value is absolute and supreme. Thus, an elderly man or woman, a mentally retarded person, a deformed baby, a dying cancer patient and similar individuals all have the same right to life as you or I. In order to preserve a human life, the Sabbath and even the Day of Atonement may be desecrated. All other rules and prohibitions, save the above three, are suspended for the overriding consideration of saving a human life.

The corollary of this principle is that one is prohibited from doing anything that might shorten a life, however briefly, since every moment of human life is also of infinite value. How does Jewish law weigh the possibility of shortening the life span of a terminally ill patient, as brief as it might be, against the possibility of cure or prolonged survival if a hazardous treatment or experimental procedure is attempted?

The problem, simply stated, is as follows: There is a patient who is extremely ill and whose prospects, under ordinary circumstances, are such that he will not live more than a very short time—perhaps only a few days or weeks. There is, however, a therapy or method available to treat that illness which, if successful, would enable the patient to recover and possibly live for a prolonged period of time. If the therapy were to prove unsuccessful, however, the patient would die immediately.

How should the physician conduct himself in such a case? Should he risk the short period of life definitely remaining to the patient by administering the drastic remedy, with the hope that perhaps the patient might be rescued from danger and live a prolonged period? In other words, should the physician abandon the *definite,* albeit short, life span of the patient in favor of the *possible* significant prolongation of his life?

This difficult problem confronts not only the physician, but the patient and his family as well. They too must be able to deal with this question, which is not purely medical. Is the patient allowed to accept hazardous surgery or experimental medical therapy? These are basic questions having medical, moral, and legal overtones. What is the view of Jewish law regarding the actions to be taken by the physician, the patient, and the family?

Let me use a case illustration to exemplify the problem:

A nine-year-old girl with acute lymphoblastic leukemia was treated with the best chemotherapeutic regimens available, yet failed to achieve remission of her disease after 8 months of treatment. Further chemotherapy had less than 5 percent chance of success. She had a very low white blood cell count and was in constant danger of developing serious and even life-threatening infection. She also had a very low platelet count and was in constant danger of serious bleeding.

The pediatric hematologists suggested bone marrow transplantation as a final resort. Tissue typing was done and the father of the child was found to have the same tissue type as the child. The chances for a successful bone marrow transplant were thought to be about 60 percent, but the procedure itself is associated with a 25 percent mortality rate and a high morbidity rate.

Most patients suffer from a complication called graft-versus-host disease in which the bone marrow donor—in this case, the father—is the cause of serious and sometimes fatal signs and symptoms in the recipient. Without the transplant, the child was thought to have no chance of remission or cure, and life expectancy was thought to be weeks or months at best. On the other hand, long-term remissions following bone marrow transplants for acute leukemia in relapse occur in perhaps 15 to 25 percent of patients.

Let us now examine the Jewish moral and ethical issues raised by this case. The child is nine years old. Does age play a role in the decision as to whether or not a bone marrow transplant is sanctioned by Jewish law? The disease afflicting the patient—acute leukemia—is, if untreated, invariably fatal. Therefore, *not* to treat seems to be an unacceptable approach in view of the supreme value of human life in Judaism. However, this patient *was* treated. The best chemotherapeutic regimens were used and were successful in arresting the disease. Now we must consider the possibility of employing the highly risky technique of bone marrow transplantation with the risk-benefit ratio cited above.

Does Judaism recognize the concept of risk-benefit ratio? Does Judaic law take into account the statistical probability of prolonging life versus the mortality rate or the odds of shortening life? May a hazardous therapeutic procedure be instituted in a dying patient if there is a slim chance of a cure, despite the fact that the chances of survival are much less than even? How does one define "slim"? Is a bone marrow transplant a recognized and accepted and widely used modality of treatment like a kidney or eye transplant, or is it still a highly experimental procedure? Does Jewish law differentiate between *therapeutic* approaches which are hazardous in nature, and hazardous procedures which are entirely experimental?

The use of drugs such as daunorubicin to treat acute leukemia is certainly fraught with hazard, since the toxicity is considerable. However, the efficacy of these and other drugs is also well known. They are able to produce long-term survival in about 50 percent of children with acute lymphoblastic leukemia. We as physicians administer these drugs in anticipation of a cure, despite the known risks. Does Judaism sanction such risks in the use of a new experimental drug or procedure whose curative potential is unknown?

In the case at hand, may the child undergo bone marrow transplantation? Must she undergo this treatment? Is bone

marrow transplantation therapeutic or experimental, or
both? May the doctor offer this form of hazardous treatment? *Must* he do so? Does Judaism have a discretionary
or mandatory attitude toward procedures which involve
significant risk? What is significant risk? Would Jewish law
sanction bone marrow transplantation in this case due to
the life-threatening nature of the underlying illness, even
though the procedure itself might lead to the early death of
the patient?

Numerous other ethical questions are involved in this
case. If the procedure is sanctioned, is consent required?
From whom? May the father subject himself to the danger
and risk, albeit small, of serving as a donor? If the child
dies following the transplant, may an autopsy be performed?

Theological and philosophical questions can also be raised
by this illustrative case. If God ordained that this child
should die at age nine of acute leukemia, how dare we interfere with God's will and attempt a bone marrow transplant to cure the child? How can we as physicians cause a
degree of harm over and above the harm associated with
the disease itself? If a physician cannot recommend a specific experimental treatment or procedure on the basis of
sound scientific principles, may he offer it as "one chance
in a million"? Would Judaism prefer an approach in which
a patient is left to chance?

The risk-benefit ratio issue is much broader than this single case illustration might lead one to believe. A seemingly
simple and straightforward subject such as immunization
against contagious diseases also involves the risk-benefit
ratio issue. There is little medical risk to the individual
undergoing immunization. There is much greater risk to the
individual and to society if immunization is *not* carried out.
Hence, such immunizations are sanctioned in Judaism, since
the small element of risk is counterbalanced by the greater
potential, as well as actual, value of the immunization.

Another area affected by the risk-benefit ratio issue is the allocation of scarce medical resources. Suppose, for example, that $1 million is available for disease prevention by screening. Should we allocate all this money, or a substantial amount of it, to screen newborns for phenylketonuria? This rare metabolic disease, if undetected and untreated, leads to profound mental retardation. Or should most or all of the money be allocated to hypertension screening programs? Hypertension is relatively common among adults and, if undetected and untreated, may be associated with stroke, heart attacks, blindness, and even death. The risk of dying is certainly much greater for the hypertensive than for the phenylketonuric. Most states, however, mandate screening of all newborn infants for phenylketonuria but do not mandate hypertension screening for adults.

Is the benefit of phenylketonuria screening to an infant, or to society, greater than the benefit to society of hypertension screening? On what basis, then, does one decide how to allocate scarce medical resources? How does one assess the risk-benefit ratio? Is the decision based—and should it be based—on considerations other than the risk or benefit to the patient? At what point do the finite resources of society loom as large as the infinite worth of human life? For the price of one B-1 bomber we could provide enough hemodialysis machines to satisfy the needs of many thousands of people who are dying of kidney failure in this country every year. Congress decided in 1973 that patients who suffer from renal disease and require dialysis have a valid claim upon the commonweal, and that available resources are therefore to be directed toward the maintenance of their viability. Medicare now pays for hemodialysis. Where may a financial line be drawn, beyond which human life will not be saved? If a hospital has six respirators, all of which are in use, and a seventh patient is admitted who requires a respirator, is the hospital obliged to purchase or rent a seventh one? One must assume that the hospital's resources are limited and finite. To remove one of the six respirators from one of the patients using it might deny that patient the possibility of recovery, and would raise a whole host of other ethical considerations relating to death and dying and euthanasia.

The final example that I would like to mention in regard to the risk-benefit ratio issue is the occurrence of leukemia and other neoplasms secondary to treatment of another cancer. Many patients who suffer one of several forms of cancer such as Hodgkin's disease, testicular cancer, breast cancer, and certain childhood cancers can now be cured with modern therapeutic approaches consisting of chemotherapy, radiation therapy, and, when appropriate, surgery. A small number of these cured patients develop acute leukemia or another malignant neoplasm many years after they have been cured of their primary cancer.

The second neoplasm—most commonly acute leukemia, which is rapidly fatal—is probably due, at least in part, to the previous anticancer drugs and/or radiation treatments which the patient received for the primary cancer. The risk of developing such a secondary neoplasm is small but genuine. The benefit of therapy to the large number of cured patients who do not develop a second neoplasm is very great indeed. The risk-benefit ratio dictates that we continue to treat and attempt to cure patients with cancer, using the standard therapeutic modalities, in spite of the risk of the later development of fatal leukemia in a small number of the cured patients.

Where the alternative—i.e., not treating the first cancer—is a 100 percent fatality rate, even a much higher risk would seem justified. But it would be inaccurate to assert that *any* risk is justified.

Returning to the case of a critically ill patient, such as the child with leukemia for whom bone marrow transplantation is being recommended, how much of a risk are the physicians morally allowed to undertake? A degree of risk is inevitable, but there are circumstances in which the doctor may actually aggravate a patient's condition or harm the patient beyond the debilitation wrought by the disease itself.

When is it ethical for a physician to employ a method which is likely to extend the life span of the patient but might result in death? To what extent is a well-intentioned physician morally culpable for the failure of an experimental procedure or some other iatrogenic complication? When the human mind is convinced that a procedure is necessary and is as free of risk as possible, should there be a "leap of faith" from animal experimentation to the experimental treatment of human patients? Should a distinction be made between hazardous standard procedures and mere experimentation?

Precise percentages cannot be used to gauge the likelihood of recovery or morbidity. In actual therapy, even a 1 percent chance of success should suffice to permit a hazardous procedure. The moral onus of omission is no less than that of commission, though Jewish law deems commission to be more severe. While no experimental procedure should be considered a "must," should the patient agree to any procedure involving even a small chance of success, even if the risks involved are greater than the potential for success? While a physician may or must offer experimental procedures when convinced that they are necessary and likely to be of help, may the patient refuse experimental treatment without violating the Jewish legal ban on suicide?

What does one do with a demented patient who refuses food, or a cancer patient who refuses hyperalimentation? To a patient with intractable pain, is death not a friend? That a terminally ill patient may request that his agony not be prolonged has its basis in the Talmud. In a famous passage *(Avodah Zarah 18a),* a distinction is implied between the deliberate termination of life and the removal of artificial means of prolonging a painful and hopeless condition. We are told of the martyrdom of Rabbi Hanina Ben Teradyon, who was a victim of the Romans during the Hadrianic persecutions of the second century. The martyr was wrapped in the Scroll of the Torah from which he had been teaching, and placed on a pyre of green brushwood. His chest was covered with woolen sponges and drenched with water to prolong the agony. His disciples advised him to open his mouth so that he might be asphyxiated and put a quicker end to his suffering. He refused to do so, saying: "It is best that He who has given life should also take it away; no one may hasten his own death."

In another Talmudic reference *(Ketubot 104a)*, the rabbis decreed a public fast and offered prayers for the prolongation of the life of the dying Rabbi Judah HaNasi. When Rabbi Judah's maid, renowned in legend for her sagacity, discerned that Rabbi Judah was terminally ill and suffering very great pain, she threw a jar from the roof to distract the rabbis and interrupt their incessant prayers. This, the Talmud says, enabled his soul to depart in peace.

While this second passage teaches that it is proper to pray that a life in suffering be ended (or at least to cease praying that it be prolonged), the first passage teaches that it is even proper to actively remove an artificial impediment to the process of dying. Accordingly, is it necessary to employ artifical means of life support in order to prolong the life of a terminally ill patient who is in agony? Is there not in Jewish law the provision *(Shulhan Arukh Yoreh De'ah 139)* which permits the removal of anything causing a hindrance to the departure of the soul of a dying person, inasmuch as such action does not involve active hastening of death but only the withdrawal of an impediment to the natural process of expiration?

Does the discontinuation of life-sustaining equipment

constitute a hastening of the patient's death—an act strictly forbidden in Judaism, which considers even a moment of life to be of infinite value? Or does the life-sustaining equipment constitute an impediment to dying which we should therefore remove?

Suppose the terminally ill patient is comatose and not suffering any pain. The psychotrauma and heavy financial burden suffered by the family may constitute agony which is no less severe for the family than physical pain may be for an individual patient. Shoudl such agony be taken into account during the treatment of the comatose patient? Or is it proper to say that where there is no patient involvement, and the patient is unable to waive any of his rights or privileges, treatment should continue?

There is another aspect to our question: When the treatment procedure is palliative rather than curative, the patient is comatose, and there is no known cure for the patient's condition, is a palliative procedure indicated? Suppose a senile patient with advanced arteriosclerosis develops appendicitis and a decision is made against performing surgery, inasmuch as the operation would be a great risk. If the patient then develops sepsis, should this latter condition be treated? Had Karen Ann Quinlan developed pneumonia, should it have been treated? Would such standard treatment for pneumonia be considered extraordinary or heroic?

It must also be said that there can be no clear, objective definition of extraordinary or heroic treatment; it differs from patient to patient. Any new treatment or any treatment beyond the basic life support systems such as feeding and washing and comforting the patient may, in some cases, be termed "heroic." In fact, medical treatment may be regarded ethically as an all-or-nothing situation, and perhaps the concept of "heroics" should not apply at all.

There is also the example of the newborn infant in a respirator, where the doctors are certain that if the infant survives it will suffer palsy or severe retardation and will be a burden on its family and on society. Should such an infant be treated to the full extent of medical knowledge and ability, or does such treatment constitute "heroics"? Should the baby just be left alone? Since a physician cannot be absolutely certain of the prognosis of an individual case, it would seem wrong to allow such discretionary latitude with regard to the suspension or termination of treatment.

I have limited my discussion to the issues of hazardous treatment, risk-benefit ratio, and life-sustaining equipment and heroic measures for the terminally ill. I have also touched briefly on the subject of "when *not* to treat." I have not discussed here the definition of death, active and passive euthanasia, "code or no code," and related issues. I have intentionally raised more questions than I have answered, and I here leave it to Rabbi Bleich to shed light on these issues from the point of view of Judaism and Jewish law.

4

Risks Versus Benefits in Treating the Gravely Ill Patient
Ethical and Religious Considerations

Rabbi J. David Bleich, Ph.D.

The pedadogic method commonly employed in teaching legal principles is known as a case method. The method is not infrequently utilized in teaching Jewish law as well. Therefore let me begin with two very real questions that were actually raised, and the answers that were given.

The first concerns a prisoner who was unjustly incarcerated and denied food and drink. He was put in jail, the door was locked, and the key thrown away. Later, some of his friends and relatives succeeded in bribing the jailer and found themselves capable of entering the jail in order to provide him with at least a minimal quantity of water and bread.

The second case involves an individual who was unjustly condemned to be burned at the stake. Again, friends and relatives succeeded in bribing the executioner. The flames were already blazing, but, in return for a fee, the executioner extinguished the fire. What degree of assistance, if any, are relatives, friends—or ordinary bystanders—obliged to extend to the prisoner in each of these cases?

One answer that was given to both of these questions is: *it all depends*—upon what one may anticipate with regard to the future. If it appears that the person in question will succeed in providing bread and water to the prisoner only on a one-time basis and that there is little or no likelihood that they will succeed in doing so in the future, then there is no obligation to do anything on behalf of the prisoner. If, however, there is reason to believe that it is possible to provide food and drink repeatedly, then there is an obligation to do so.

There is one question, and one question only, which must be resolved: our attitude toward the preservation of life. I speak of the "preservation of life" not so much as a value in and of itself, but as a relative value. After all, who doesn't subscribe to the principle that life is good and sacred and that one ought to go to great lengths in order to preserve life? The question is, what value is to be assigned to human life when preservation of human life comes into conflict with *other* values? Is preservation of human life an absolute value? Or is preservation of human life—while a significant value, to be sure—not a paramount or transcendental value, but merely one value among many.

Let me give you one example in Western literature which makes this point in a very dramatic way. Everyone is familiar with the Robin Hood story. Like many others, I read Robin Hood as a child. Years later, I found myself vicariously rereading Robin Hood together with my children. But the Robin Hood narrative with which I became acquainted as an adult seems to me quite different from the Robin Hood that I read as a child. On the second reading I discovered that Robin Hood is a philosophical treatise which a professor of ethics might assign as required reading without hesitation or embarrassment because it presents, in a concrete way, an acute moral dilemma.

Everybody remembers the facts. Robin Hood robs the Sheriff of Nottingham and other personages of rank and affluence. However, he robs them not for purposes of self-enrichment, but in order to feed starving widows and orphans. The Sheriff of Nottingham is outraged that his material possessions be expropriated for this purpose even though his wealth is to be used to save lives of individuals who would otherwise die.

In stating that there is a great deal that can be said for the position espoused by the Sheriff of Nottingham, I am not playing devil's advocate. We are confronted by two values which, in this situation, come into harsh conflict. Everyone subscribes to a moral code. Every civilized person subscribes to a value system in which "Thou shalt not kill" occupies a central position, and the corollary of "Thou shalt not kill" is "Thou shalt not stand idly by the blood of thy fellow." Certainly every civilized person also recognizes that every individual must respect the inviolability of property belonging to his neighbor. After all, "Thou shalt not steal" is also a biblical commandment. But what happens when "Thou shalt not steal" comes into conflict with "Thou shalt not kill" or "Thou shalt not stand idly by the blood of thy fellow"?

In every value system, and hence in every ethical and moral system, it is not sufficient simply to posit a certain set of values. It is not enough simply to catalogue the ideals by which men choose to guide their lives. In addition to a statement of values to be adopted, there must also be either a hierarchical ranking of those values or else a set of rules or canons to be applied in determining how an individual is to conduct himself when those values come into conflict. With regard to any value system one must ask whether respect for the property rights of another is to be given priority over preservation of life, or whether preservation of life is a paramount value to which all other values are to be deemed subservient.

The Sheriff of Nottingham obviously resolves this moral dilemma in his own way. For him, respect for property rights—"Thou shalt not steal"—constitutes the dominant value. For Robin Hood, the preservation of human life takes precedence over respect for the property rights of others. And it will be remembered that in Robin Hood's band was an individual by the name of Friar Tuck—actually, a professor of Moral Theology. His role is to give ecclesiastic endorsement to the choice made by Robin Hood. And it can be said that Jewish law reflects the same hierarchical ranking of values. In fact, when the question is put in such crass material terms, every moral individual would recognize that Robin Hood was justified in appropriating the equivalent of a few loaves of bread from the vast resources of the Sheriff of Nottinghan in order to save the lives of starving orphans and widows.

In our society, the dilemma is posed in somewhat different terms. As a result we react, at times, not as Robin Hood reacted, but as did the Sheriff of Nottingham. The American Declaration of Independence espouses certain "inalienable rights," a phrase synonymous with philosophers' principles of natural law. The underlying notion is that every man is created by God and endowed by Him with certain liberties and prerogatives which cannot be alienated from him. Those are, in the eyes of our Founding Fathers, "life, liberty, and the pursuit of happiness." In the philosophy of John Locke this notion was phrased a little bit differently: Locke spoke of life, liberty, and enjoyment of property. To the American mind, the concept of happiness is, quite evidently, reducible to enjoyment of property. The "inalienable rights" of which the Declaration of Independence speaks represent fundamental values. Individuals are endowed with life, and have a God-given right to have that life safeguarded and protected. Individuals are endowed with liberty, and no one ought to interfere with the personal autonomy of any other human being. Individuals are entitled to the pursuit of happiness and to the undisturbed enjoyment of their property.

But does it therefore follow that an individual has the right to commit suicide? Does an individual have the right to demand that his physician withhold life-saving therapy? What happens when the right to liberty, the right of personal autonomy, comes into conflict with the value of preservation of life? Or, in dealing with the third element in our triad, what happens when the value known as preservation of life comes into conflict either with happiness or with its analogue, preservation of property?

After all, society possesses only a finite amount of material resources, or so we are told. What happens when preservation of life simply costs too much? Preservation of life may be deemed to cost too much in terms of the expenditure of resources and services in prolonging that life, or it may cost too much in emotional coin because the patient is in pain, the family is in a state of anguish, and the physicians experience frustration because, their diligent ministrations notwithstanding, they are incapable of effecting a cure. What happens when a conflict arises between preservation of life and promotion of happiness by means of elimination of pain? Happiness and elimination of pain are, after all, but two sides of the same coin. In the real world such values often come into conflict.

Well-intentioned individuals may differ with regard to the

proper resolution of such dilemmas. Different moral traditions have certainly presented diverse answers. The Catholic tradition asserts that preservation of life is but one value among many. But Jewish tradition teaches that preservation of life is of paramount value and that virtually all other values are rendered subservient to the overriding value of preservation of human life.

It is for that reason that Jewish ethics could not possibly countenance a "no-code" directive routinely entered on the charts of certain categories of patients. There may be very limited circumstances in which treatment may be withheld, but certainly a decision to withhold treatment cannot be made in an across-the-board or arbitrary manner. Indeed, insofar as Judaism is concerned, such a decision can be made only upon consultation with a knowledgeable rabbinic authority. Life and death decisions have to be made on a case-by-case basis and any general rule should only be used as a guideline.

The question is often posed: Is it worthwhile to preserve the life of an individual if that life is going to be fraught with excruciating pain? Is preservation of the life of an individual desirable if the individual is going to live the life of a human vegetable?

There is one axiological point which must be recognized in order to understand the Jewish answer to these questions as well as to so many related questions. In Judaism, the preservation of life takes precedence over virtually all ritual commandments and assuredly takes precedence over virtually any other concern and any other consideration. Life is of infinite value; indeed, every moment of life is of infinite value. Questions regarding the *quality* of the life which is to be preserved are of no direct relevance in determining whether therapeutic procedures should or should not be instituted or whether life-support systems should or should not be withheld or withdrawn.

The question of extending a life fraught with pain versus allowing the patient to die is one which the sages of the Gemara addressed, and addressed very forthrightly. They spoke of an individual who was liable to the punishment of death at the hands of Heaven. They made a point of demonstrating, on the basis of the Talmudic interpretation of biblical passages, that an individual in such a situation may, by virtue of earned merit, receive a certain mitigation of that punishment. And what is the mitigation of punishment? Instead of death, the punishment is of a nature that I can only describe as a form of excruciating agony. It is extremely significant that the sages of the Talmud spoke of this mitigated punishment as something which an individual earns on the basis of merit and which is bestowed by God Himself as an act of grace. Thus, Jewish tradition clearly recognizes that life accompanied by pain is, in a certain profound sense, preferable to death. But at the same time, it recognizes that an individual suffering from an illness fraught with pain has an absolute right to address himself to God through prayer and to beseech of God that the life which has become too burdensome be taken away from him.

There is a remarkable statement by Rabbenu Nissim Gerondi, a fourteenth-century talmudic commentator, which defines the *mitzvah* of *bikkur cholim,* the commandment concerning visitation of the sick. *Bikkur cholim* is a *mitzvah* everybody knows about. It is a popular *mitzvah;* it is, or appears to be, an easy *mitzvah* to fulfill. One spends a few moments in social chitchat and one has earned a good deed into the bargain. But spending a few minutes with a patient does not necessarily, in and of itself, constitute the fulfillment of a commandment. The *mitzvah* of *bikkur cholim,* as defined by Rabbenu Nissim, requires that a *service* be performed on behalf of the patient.

In the days when there were no medical centers or nursing homes and, other than physicians, no health care professionals, friends and family had to come and provide food, feed and bathe the patient, and perform other personal services. Today we have institutionalized almost every aspect of human life and we have professionals who perform the services which constitute the essence of the *mitzvah* of *bikkur cholim*. What, then, is left for an ordinary friend to do?

Certainly, if a patient derives pleasure from a friend's visit and this somehow mitigates his pain and mental anguish, then the firend has performed a personal service and has earned a *mitzvah*. But no matter what the situation may be, declares Rabbenu Nissim, a visitor can always perform a *mitzvah*. There is one way in which every visitor can fulfill the commandment of *bikkur cholim;* there is one thing that the patient can not get enough of, and that is called prayer. Prayer is a distinct service which any and every person can perform on behalf of the patient.

Now, this thesis appears to be unexceptionable. Rabbenu Nissim, however, goes on to say that, while in most cases the prayer is for the *cure* of the patient, in other situations the prayer may be addressed to God beseeching Him to put an end to the patient's misery. Not only is such prayer entirely permissible, declares Rabbenu Nissim, but such a prayer actually constitutes the fulfillment of the biblical commandment of *bikkur cholim*. This, too, is a service performed on behalf of the sick.

There is a world of difference between recognition that at times life is a burden, and failing to fulfill one's obligation with regard to preservation of that life. Jewish law provides, for example, that Sabbath restrictions may be violated on behalf of a dangerously ill individual without in any way qualifying that provision with regard to the quality of the life which is preserved. Sabbath restrictions, as well as other provisions of Jewish law, are waived—indeed, under such circumstances it is mandatory that such restrictions be ignored—in order to preserve the life of an individual who is insane, in order to preserve the life of an individual who is a "vegetable," and to preserve or prolong the life of a comatose patient. The *quality* of life preserved is of no consideration whatsoever in tempering the obligation to preserve and to prolong life, even when the requisite action would ordinarily be regarded as a violation of Jewish law.

The question is, why? What does all of this mean? What is the underlying rationale? I think that the basic concept is best expressed by Rabbi David ibn Zimra (Radvaz), the author of one of the standard commentaries on Maimonides' *Mishneh Torah*, who formulates his thesis by drawing attention to what appears to be a contradiction between two fundamental principles of Jewish law.

There is a principle of Jewish jurisprudence which provides that an individual may appear before a *Bet Din* and make a statement which is prejudicial to his own financial interests and the statement will be accepted without question and without qualification. This is true even if the statement is contradicted by the testimony of a hundred trustworthy and credible witnesses. For example, Mr. A may appear in court and say, "I have borrowed $100 from Mr. B on such and such a day and I have not returned the money." The *Bet Din* will order him to return the money even if a hundred witnesses appear and testify that the story of the loan is a complete fabrication.

Yet, with regard to criminal procedure, Jewish law contains a provision which goes far beyond the Fifth Amendment. The Fifth Amendment says simply that an individual cannot be compelled to give testimony against himself. Nevertheless, confessions of guilt are not barred and, indeed, are commonly accepted by our courts. Jewish law declares that not only can a witness not be compelled to testify against himself, but that, in criminal matters, any statement which is prejudicial to the interests of the defendant is inadmissible if the statement comes from the mouth of the defendant. No individual can be convicted on the basis of his own testimony and no individual is accorded credence in declaring himself to be a criminal.

Radvaz' problem lies in the obvious contradiction presented by these two rules. Either a person is to be granted credence with regard to statements prejudicial to his own interest or he is to be regarded as lacking credibility with regard to his own deeds. If his statements are to be given weight, they should be given the same weight in criminal matters as they are given in matters of jurisprudence. On the other hand, if statements made by an individual are regarded as untrustworthy and unreliable insofar as they pertain to himself and to his own interests, such statements should be dismissed out of hand in civil proceedings just as they are in criminal matters.

The answer, as Radvaz phrases it, is really very simple. After all, observes Radvaz, an individual's material possessions and financial resources are his to dispose of as he wishes. A person's money is his own. If he wishes, he is at perfect liberty to make a gift of his funds to another person. If he chooses to invoke the judicial process as an instrument in accomplishing that end, the law will be happy to accommodate him. It may be nothing more than a charade, but there is more than one way to skin a cat and more than one way to bestow a gift. Accordingly, if a person wishes to make a gift by harnessing the judicial process in order to do so, so be it. However, an individual who is prosecuted on criminal charges and who, if found guilty, is subject to either corporal or capital punishment, in confessing guilt, is not giving away his money but is disposing of his body and his life. But man's body and his life are not his to give away. Judaism teaches man has no proprietary interest either in his life or in his body. The proprietor of all of human life is none other than God Himself. As Radvaz so eloquently phrases it: "Man's life is not his property, but the property of the Holy One, blessed be He."

And what is the status of the legal relationship which exists between man and his body? In order to understand Jewish teaching with regard to the various problems that were raised earlier, it is necessary to draw a kind of analogy. We must recognize that personal privilege as well as personal responsibility, as it extends to the human body and to human life, is similar to the privilege and responsibility of a bailee with regard to a bailment with which he has been entrusted.

A bailee is an individual who has accepted an object of value for safekeeping. The nature of the regulations governing the responsibilities of a bailee differs from the nature of Jewish law as it pertains to other areas of responsibility. Perhaps an example will best illustrate the point.

The Gemara, *Baba Batra* 23b, establishes a rule with regard to ownership of doves or pigeons. If a person comes upon a pigeon in a field and wants to take the pigeon for himself and if the pigeon is *hefker,* ownerless or abandoned, then, of course, "finders, keepers." Anyone who finds such a pigeon can acquire title simply by taking the pigeon into his possession. If, however, the pigeon is the property of another person the finder may not take the pigeon for himself—to do so would be theft. Quite to the contrary, an individual who finds lost property is under obligation to restore it to its rightful owner.

But how does one determine whether the pigeon is ownerless property or whether it has merely wandered off from its coop? The Mishnah establishes a rule. It declares that if a dove is found in the immediate vicinity of a pigeon coop, it must be presumed that it belongs to the owner of the pigeon coop. If there is no pigeon coop in the immediate vicinity, it may be assumed that the pigeon has no owner and, accordingly, the finder may take possession of the pigeon and do with it as he wishes. But of course, it is necessary to define what is meant by the immediate vicinity of a pigeon coop. The Mishnah states that if the pigeon is found within 50 cubits of the coop—that is, within 75 feet or 100 feet, depending upon how a cubit is to be measured—it belongs to the owner of the pigeon coop. If the pigeon is found more than 50 cubits away from the coop it belongs to the finder.

The Gemara relates that along came a scholar by the name of Rabbi Jeremiah and posed the following question: What if the pigeon, when it is found, is found standing with one foot within the 50-cubit limit and one foot outside the 50-cubit limit? We don't find an answer in the pages of the Gemara. Instead the Gemara tells us that for asking that question Rabbi Jeremiah was expelled from the academy.

That is certainly extraordinary. We teach our students that every question must be taken seriously and that every question deserves an answer. But here we seem to be confronted with a case which contradicts that principle. Why didn't Rabbi Jeremiah receive an answer? His question was entirely cogent and certainly deserved serious consideration.

Tosafot explains why Rabbi Jeremiah did not receive an answer. *Tosafot* explains that Rabbi Jeremiah was expelled from the House of Study, not because he asked a foolish question and not because the question was audacious. The 50 cubit rule, very precisely formulated by the Mishnah, is founded upon the premise that a pigeon will not, under any circumstances, wander a greater distance from its coop. The pigeon may stray up to 50 cubits but not one millimeter beyond. If the principle is that a pigeon cannot or will not hop, skip, jump, or fly more than 50 cubits, then if it is found with one foot beyond the 50 cubits limit, it could not possibly have come from the pigeon coop. Since the rule is formulated so precisely, a pigeon found under such circumstances must be deemed ownerless and becomes the finder's property.

Rabbi Jeremiah was expelled from the academy, not because he asked bothersome questions, but because he was found lacking in the requirements for admission. He was found lacking because he didn't recognize that Jewish law adheres to what contemporary scholars call legal formalism. In common law, the system of law followed in the United States, most questions of fact which are subject to dispute are resolved by applying a "reasonable man" formula. If it is necessary to know how to interpret a certain event, or how to analyze the text of an ambiguous document, or what obligations a person has assumed in a certain situation, the matter is presented to a jury and the jury determines the view a "reasonable man" would take with regard to the facts under dispute. In such a system of law there are seldom hard and fast rules which apply to all situations. The "reasonable man" makes determinations within the context of the many variables of any particular situation.

Jewish law is quite different and the reason for the difference is very simple. As a late justice of the Israeli Supreme Court, Moshe Silberg, has pointed out, Jewish law is based primarily on the concept of *duty,* as distinct from the concept of *right.* If one goes to a lawyer and solicits his advice with regard to a specific matter—shall I or shall I not take a certain deduction on my income tax return, shall I or shall I not draft a contract in a certain way—the lawyer will respond by saying, "Well, let's see what would happen if the matter becomes the subject of litigation. How is the jury likely to react?"

A Jew who places a similar question before a halakhic authority is not concerned with possible punishment or financial liability; he is primarily concerned with determining moral obligations. Moral obligations, as distinct from legal rights, must be precise. If, for example, a person comes to ask whether something is kosher or nonkosher, his inquiry concerns a matter of religious obligation and the answer must be clearcut and precise. He must determine without equivocation whether a certain act is permitted or forbidden. Similarly, an inquiry with regard to property rights or financial considerations is a question with regard to the propriety of a certain course of action, not a question regarding possible liability. Hence the answer must be clearcut and precise. An answer is required before the action is carried out and cannot abide the determination of a jury with regard to how a "reasonable man" would perceive the situation. Therefore Jewish law must employ rules which can be applied in a categorical and formal manner. It is because it employs such inelastic rules that Jewish law is often categorized as excessively formalistic, and often in a derogatory sense. However, if one bears in mind that Judaism is concerned first and foremost with assessment of *obligation,* it is understandable that objective standards must be immediately available in order to enable people to regulate their conduct.

It turns out, however, that a major exception to the formalism which is the hallmark of Jewish law lies in the area of medicine and bioethics. Here we find problems which lend themselves to multiple answers, situations in which there is room for discretion. These are situations in which the answer is not automatically yes or no, but in which the answer can be yes, no, or maybe, and all three answers may conceivably be correct. The reason for this is, I believe, as has been indicated earlier, that the situation is one involving obligations analogous to those of a bailee.

Human life and the human body are given to man for safekeeping. Man is entrusted with the preservation of his life and the protection of his body. Man is given the responsibility of caring for his body, of nurturing it, and of preserving its health. It is not always clear how these ends can best be advanced. At times, a person must make choices and the proper choice is not always obvious. Similarly, a bailee must safeguard and preserve the property which has been entrusted to him for safekeeping. Here too the rule, in its theory, is clear enough. But, in application, it is not always obvious what specific course of action will yield the desired result. No system of law could possible envisage every possible contingency and provide a specific a priori rule to be applied in every conceivable situation. This is certainly true with regard to treatment of sickness and disease.

The most obvious and, for our purposes, the most suitable example which serves to illustrate this point is the question of whether or not there exists an obligation to treat, and to seek treatment, when the only available therapy involves a procedure that is hazardous in nature. There is, to be sure, a general obligation to treat. The obligation to treat is part of the broader obligation to preserve life. But, whenever one treats a patient, whenever one attempts to preserve the life of a patient, one, almost by definition, endangers the life of the patient. Nachmanides, writing in the thirteenth century, put it beautifully: "There is no medicine that is capable of curing one patient which cannot at the same time kill another patient." If a medicine is sufficiently potent to be of use pharmacologically it is potent enough to do damage as well. This means, then, that the obligation to treat is at one and the same time also a dispensation to assume certain risks. A problem arises because at a certain point the risks, relative to the possible benefits that may be realized, are simply too great to be prudently undertaken.

In the value system reflected in Jewish law and ethics, the risk/benefit dilemma arises when the treatment carries with it the risk of foreshortening what remains of the natural life span of the patient. There is little question that an otherwise terminally ill patient should be given radiation therapy, if medically indicated, even though the radiation may result in leukemia several decades later. But a dilemma does arise in the case of a patient who, if left untreated, will live for days or weeks or even months, but who, if treated, will either experience a complete recovery and live out his allotted span of years or, if the therapy is not successful, will have his life foreshortened and die earlier than had he not been treated.

It is, of course, necessary to pinpoint the threshold of danger beyond which a therapeutic procedure is deemed hazardous. Obviously, administering an aspirin under normal circumstances is not to be classified as hazardous, although in some rare instances complications may well arise as a result of aspirin therapy. By the same token, if the patient is not known to be allergic, administration of penicillin for the treatment of pneumonia would not be considered a hazardous procedure. In these and similar cases there may well exist certain dangers. Nevertheless, those risks are minimal and well below the threshold of significant danger. There are, however, situations in which the therapy is indeed hazardous in nature. In such cases employment of a hazardous therapy is discretionary. The decision to employ such procedures requires a careful analysis of the risk/benefit ratio, i.e., an analysis of the possibility of longevity enhancement as opposed to possible diminution of life expectancy. It is the patient who is charged with safeguarding and preserving the life with which he has been entrusted who has the right and the responsibility for making such decisions.

Of course, such decisions must be informed and shaped by the relevant provisions of Jewish law. The patient who consults his rabbi before making a decision does so because he is confronted by a moral and halakhic problem and is in need of expert advice in determining a proper cause of action, just as he requires expert advice from his physician in establishing the parameters within which this moral decision must be made. In some situations the risk/benefit ratio may leave little room for discretion. In others, the judgment call may be extremely difficult. But, ultimately, it is the patient who must make the determination with regard to the prudent course, just as a bailee must often exercise discretion with regard to how best to preserve the property which has been entrusted to him for safekeeping.

An individual charged with safeguarding and preserving property entrusted to him may legitimately assume certain risks, since, if he fails to take the risk, the property may be totally destroyed. On the other hand, the selfsame measures which he takes in order to assure the preservation of that which has been entrusted to him may instead contribute in loss or diminution in the value of the bailment. Similarly, the patient making a decision with regard to utilization of hazardous therapy is, in effect, deciding how he can best preserve the bailment which has been committed to him for safekeeping. In a like manner, Jewish law recognizes that, when the patient is incapable of making a reasoned decision, the next of kin, or the person charged with supervising the affairs of the patient and who serves, in effect, as the guardian of the patient, must make such decisions on behalf of the patient.

It must, however, be added that, although informed consent must be obtained prior to instituting hazardous procedures, Jewish law recognizes no such requirement with regard to other standard forms of treatment. Jewish law, unlike common law, does not at all demand that a patient consent to a procedure designed to restore health or to prolong life. On the contrary, Jewish law demands that the patient seek medical advice and that he submit to the ministrations of the physician. The physician is under divine mandate to treat and the patient is under equal obligation to accept treatment, provided that the treatment itself is not hazardous in nature.

Experimental procedures similarly fall into the category of discretionary measures even though the experimental procedure in question may be nonhazardous. An individual has an obligation to preserve life. The limitations placed upon the obligation of the bailee are that he safeguard and preserve the property entrusted to him in a manner in which a reasonable man would exercise vigilance and care. An individual's obligation with regard to his life and health are likewise limited to the exercise of vigilance and care in a customary and usual manner—in a way in which people in general customarily preserve life and health. Experimental procedures, while not forbidden, certainly are not customary and usual and hence are not mandatory.

This is at best but a broad sketch of the philosophical perspective of Judaism with regard to treatment of the ill. But surely one basic principle emerges with some degree of clarity: namely, that Jewish tradition manifests an unabashed bias in favor of life and a pronounced predisposition to treat the sick by means of any mode of therapy which may be available. To paraphrase an eloquent comment of Judge Skelly Wright appended to a classic decision in a case involving a question of this nature: "It may very well be that I have erred; but if to err, I prefer to err on the side of life."

5

Filial Responsibility to the "Senile" Parent
A Jewish Approach

Rabbi Levi Meier, Ph.D.

The guidelines for interpersonal relations which cover life-cycle situations are a distinct aspect of Jewish law. For example, comforting the bereaved requires the comforter to be completely silent until the bereaved begins a conversation (Karo, *Shulhan Arukh, Yoreh Deah,* 376.1). Similarly, the laws for visiting the sick require certain behavior, such as saying words of encouragement and helping the sick to arrange their financial affairs (*ibid.,* 335.7).

Under ordinary circumstances the behavior required for honoring one's father and mother is conceptually defined by two categories: honor *(kibbud)* and reverence *(morah)*. *Honor* is defined as positive acts of personal service. Rabbinic examples include feeding and dressing one's parent (Talmud, *Kiddushin,* 31b). These examples illustrate that a child's relationship to the parent is comparable to that of a servant to the master. *Reverence* is defined as an avoidance of disrespectful acts. Rabbinic examples include not sitting in a parent's seat nor speaking before parents and never contradicting them (Talmud, *Kiddushin,* 31b). These examples demonstrate how, in general, a child should relate to superiors.

These child-parent obligations are applicable throughout the life cycle; when the parents are young, middle-aged, and in the late period of life. The purpose of this chapter is to analyze whether these obligations are similarly applicable when one's parent is senile.

"Senility" does not refer to forgetfulness or excessive reminiscing on the part of the aged parent. Senility, which is irreversible, is defined as chronic brain syndrome (Butler & Lewis, 1973). Acute brain syndrome is reversible and does not fall in the category of senility. The mental status questionnaire devised by Kahn, Goldfarb, Pollack, and Peck (1960) clearly differentiates between acute and chronic brain syndrome.

Acute brain syndrome (ABS) differs from chronic brain syndrome in the areas of causes, symptoms, and treatment. For purposes of this discussion, symptoms and treatment are the most significant considerations. Reversible brain syndrome involves a fluctuating level of awareness. The person typically is disoriented; recent memory is lost, while remote memory may be preserved. Restlessness or aggressiveness may appear in the behavior (Butler & Lewis, 1973; Libow, 1973; Verwoerdt, 1976).

The clinical symptoms of chronic brain syndrome (CBS) differ significantly from those of reversible brain syndrome. There are two predominant types of chronic brain syndrome: *senile psychosis* and *psychosis associated with cerebral arteriosclerosis.*

The symptoms of *senile psychosis* may appear insidiously without any abrupt changes. Gradually, small differences in physical, mental, and emotional functioning are noticed. Early symptoms may include errors in judgment and decline in personal care and habits. Depression, anxiety, and irritability may also characterize the early stages of this syndrome. As the deterioration increases, the traditional five signs of organic dysfunction become more evident: (1) disturbance and impairment of memory; (2) impairment of intellectual functioning; (3) impairment of judgment; (4) impairment of orientation, and (5) shallow or labile affect.

The symptoms of *psychosis associated with cerebral arteriosclerosis* can either be gradual or sudden. With a slower onset, there is usually a gradual intellectual loss, and impairment of memory tends to be spotty rather than complete. The course is up and down rather than progressively downhill (Butler & Lewis, 1973; Verwoerdt, 1976).

It appears that the reversible brain syndrome can result in complete recovery once the person survives the physical crises which precipitated the psychiatric disorder. Treatment must be intensive but can often be short-term.

Senile psychosis is marked by steady and progressive deterioration and is eventually fatal. Emotional reactions may respond to treatment, and physical functioning can improve with proper support even though the physical loss is irreparable. Similarly, psychosis associated with cerebral arteriosclerosis can lead quickly to a fatal outcome or may produce an organic condition lasting a number of years.

The salient differences between chronic and acute brain syndrome are well documented by Kay (1972).

In attempting to arrive at the Jewish law regarding care of a senile parent, one must rely not only on scientific definitions of brain syndromes, but also on the Talmudic treatment of mental dysfunction in a parent. An examination of pertinent Talmudic passages may be instructive in attempting to ascertain the *halakhic* differentiation between abnormal behavior and mental disturbance as well as the required behavior under Jewish law for dealing with one's senile parent.

The Talmud asks the question, "How far does the honor of parents extend?" (Talmud, *Kiddushin,* 31a). A few Talmudic anecdotes would appear to indicate that if a parent behaves abnormally, the child's responsibility to honor the father or mother is not altered. Rabbi Dimi gives this incident as an example:

> Once he [Dama the son of Metinah] was seated among the great men of Rome, dressed in a gold embroidered, silk garment, when his mother came and tore the garment from him, slapped him on the head, and spat in his face—but he did not shame her (Talmud, *Kiddushin,* 31a).

Rabbi Eliezer further asserts that even should the parent take the child's purse, and, in the child's presence, throw the purse into the sea, the child must still not shame the parent (*ibid.,* 32a).

These citations illustrate that even extreme deviations from normal parental behavior in no way alter the child's obligation to honor the parent, which remains an absolute, no matter what the difficulties of the child.

Maimonides codifies the two foregoing examples and establishes normative principles to guide people faced with similar circumstances:

> How far must one go to honor one's father and mother? Even if they took his wallet full of gold pieces and threw it into the sea before his very eyes, he must not shame them, show pain before them or display anger to them; but he must accept the decree of scripture and keep his silence. And how far must one go in reverence? Even if he is dressed in precious clothes and is sitting in an honored place before many people, and his parents come and tear his clothes, hitting him in the head and

spitting in his face, he may not shame them, but he must keep silent, and be in awe and fear of the King of Kings who commanded him thus. For if a king of flesh and blood had decreed that he do something more painful than this, he could not hesitate in its performance. How much more so, when he is commanded by Him who created the world at His will (Maimonides, *Mishneh Torah*, Laws of Mamrim [the Rebellious], 6.7).

Maimonides realizes the difficulties inherent in these events and in implementing these commandments. In his view, an additional motivation for the performance of these commandments stems from one's awe and fear of the King of Kings.

From these Talmudic anecdotes and from Maimonides' analysis of them, it would appear, as previously assumed, that if a parent behaves abnormally, the child's responsibility to honor the father or mother is not altered. On the contrary, one finds that the child's responsibility increases in direct proportion to the specific needs of the parents. Also, as at any other time, personal service (honor) and the avoidance of disrespect (reverence) must characterize dealings with a parent in such a situation.

However, in addition to the codification of these two examples, Maimonides establishes a separate category for the conduct required in dealing with one's *mentally disturbed* parent. Maimonides writes:

If one's father or mother should become mentally disordered, he should try to treat them as their mental state demands, until they are pitied [by God]. But if he finds he cannot endure the situation because of their extreme madness, let him leave and go away, assigning others to care for them properly (*Mishneh Torah*, Laws of Mamrim, 6.10).

Though there is no specific Talmudic statement upon which this view of Maimonides is based, the commentaries on Maimonides assume that the following anecdote is the basis for his statement:

> Rabbi Assi had an aged mother. Said she to him, "I want ornaments." So he made them for her. . . . "I want a husband as handsome as you." Thereupon he left her and went to Palestine (Talmud, *Kiddushin,* 31b).

The departure of Rabbi Assi from Babylon has been interpreted as an acceptable response to the action of his senile mother. Rabbi Assi, unable to respond to his aged, senile mother in a constructive manner, leaves her in Babylon and makes his way to Palestine.

Maimonides clearly does more than just codify this Talmudic event. He adds some interpretive dimensions. His codification accentuates three essential points, as Blidstein (1975) points out:

1. The parent is classified as mentally disturbed.
2. The child is exempt from personal service to the parent, but not from the responsibility to ensure that others attend to the parent.
3. The point of the child's exemption from personal service to the senile parent is the child's own evaluation of the situation.

The Rabad argues with Maimonides' conclusion. He asks, "If he leaves, whom will he assign to watch his parents?" (*Mishneh Torah,* Laws of Mamrin, 6.10).

In Rabad's view, there is no limitation to the child's responsibility. Instructive here is the defense of Maimonides' view offered by Radvaz (*Mishneh Torah,* Laws of Mamrim, 6.10), who claims that the child is in a weakened position, unable to rebuke the parent and not able to command the respect necessary to effect some measure of stability. An outsider is unencumbered by these realities and is better able to restore the parent to a more functional level. The child's exemption from service to the parent is thus a perceptive clinical judgment.

The basic question arising from Maimonides' citations centers on his differentiation between a parent's acting abnormally and being mentally disturbed. Abnormal parental behavior must be withstood by the child, but care of a mentally disturbed parent may be delegated to others.

The examples of parental behavior given by the Talmud—throwing the son's wallet into the sea and tearing his clothes in front of dignitaries, in contrast to saying, "I want a husband as handsome as you"—are not, in themselves, sufficient for differentiating between abnormal behavior and mental disturbance.

The key issue in these situations is the halakhically acceptable response to these problems. The son must tolerate abnormal parental behavior, even abuse. However, Rabbi Assi, whose mother desired a husband as handsome as he, is allowed to depart for Palestine, leaving care of his aged mother to others.

One suggested explanation for these two distinct *halakhic* codifications by Maimonides may be that he equates Rabbi Assi's mother's condition with chronic, irreversible brain syndrome, while he regards the examples of parental abuse as cases of temporary abnormality.

According to Jewish law, the categories of *honor* and *reverence* apply in the cases of every normal and abnormal parent behavior, but *honor* may be suspended in cases of behavior which result from permanent mental disturbance. Even extreme deviations from the norm and totally illogical behavior on the part of parents must be tolerated when that behavior is the result of an acute condition, such as an acute brain syndrome. In these cases, filial responsibility increases according to parental needs and constructive responses can be expected, since the situation is reversible.

However, a chronic brain syndrome, an irreversible condition, falls into a different category. It is recognized that the child's tolerance may be overtaxed and the child is therefore exempted from direct personal service. However, the responsibility to ensure that someone else takes care of the parent is incumbent upon the child.

This hypothesis concerning the differentiation between acute and chronic brain syndrome in determining the applicable Jewish law is hinted at by Maimonides when he asserts that the child must try to treat the parent as the mental state demands, but if enduring the situation is no longer possible because the madness is extreme (chronic), the child *should* leave and assign others to care for the parent (*Mishneh Torah,* Laws of Mamrim, 6.10). That is, every mental disturbance must be initially dealt with until filial tolerance is exhausted due to the parent's extreme condition. This condition must be chronic and therefore, irreversible. An acute brain syndrome, although very taxing, will not worsen, but will indeed improve significantly when dealt with. In such a situation, filial responsibility is not suspended.

With an understanding of the distinction between these two types of brain syndrome, different filial responses toward abnormal parental behavior may be understood. Naturally, every deviation from the parental norm must initially be treated as acute until evidence indicates that the condition is in fact irreversible. Chronic brain syndrome may be a legitimate reason for transferring the obligation for attentiveness to a parent's needs to others. However, old age and the normal infirmities that may accompany it do not provide sufficient reason for transferring this obligation. Old age is expected to stimulate additional contact between parent and offspring rather than abandonment of the parent.

REFERENCES

Blidstein, G. *Honor thy father and mother: Filial responsibility in Jewish law and ethics.* New York: KTAV Publishing House, Inc., Yeshiva University Press, 1975

Butler, R.N., & Lewis, M.I. *Aging and mental health.* St. Louis: C.V. Mosby Company, 1973.

Kahn, R.L., Goldfarb, A.L., Pollack, M., & Peck A. Brief objective measures for the determination of mental status in the aged. *American Journal of Psychiatry,* 1960, *117*(4), 326-328.

Karo, J. *Shulchan Arukh* (10 vols.). New York: M.P. Press, 1965.

Kay, D.W.K. Epidemiological aspects of organic brain disease in the aged. In C.M. Gaitz (Ed.), *Aging and the brain.* New York: Plenum Press, 1972.

Libow, L.S. Pseudo-senility: Acute and reversible organic brain syndromes. *Journal of the American Geriatrics Society.* 1973, *21*(3), 12-120.

Maimonides, M. *Mishneh Torah* (6 vols). New York: M.P. Press, 1962.

Verwoerdt, A. *Clinical geropsychiatry.* Baltimore: Williams and Wilkins, 1976.

6

Ethical Problems Regarding the Termination of Life

Sir Immanuel Jakobovits, Ph.D.

In dealing with a number of specific issues, I will first attempt to offer a glimpse into what might be termed the modus operandi of Jewish law. How does Jewish law go to work in relating to very modern issues, many of which obviously are the result of spectacular advances in medicine that are of very recent times? How can we apply to contemporary perplexities insights that have their origin in the timeless traditions of our faith and are imbedded in virtually all the layers of our literature going back to earliest biblical times? How we can find principles enshrined in those early sources that have relevance and application to the highly complex questions that arise from these dramatic advances in medicine? Such advances are most notable in the past half century, when we have witnessed a virtual knowledge explosion in the field of medicine, as indeed in other sciences.

The first subject I was asked to discuss provides a classic example of how we can utilize earlier antecedents for the solution of present-day problems. That is the question of informing patients of their medical condition: to tell or not to tell.

This, I am sure, is a problem that troubles and challenges not only every physician in his routine practice, but which he very often has to share with the families of patients who are deeply exercised by this problem. Should we or should we not inform the patient of a fatal diagnosis that may have been made? Or, to put it more bluntly, if he were to put the straightforward question to the doctor—"Do I have cancer, or don't I?"—do you or don't you tell him?

Interestingly enough, there is perhaps no area in the widely ramified field of Jewish medical ethics that provides a more striking example of how we may use an ancient source to resolve a current moral dilemma. It is not necessary to go to all the more recent rabbinic responsa, or to the rabbinic law codifications, or even to the Talmud. We find direct precedent in the Bible that served later generations of rabbis as a definition of our attitude to this very problem of "to tell or not to tell."

The Book of Kings relates the story of a Syrian king, Ben Haddad, who was gravely ill. He wanted to know whether he would live, or succumb to his disease. He sent a messenger named Chazael to the land of Israel, to consult Elisha, the prophet. Elisha said to the messenger, "Tell the king he will surely live." Then he added, "Albeit I know that he will surely die." Thus Elisha, a man inspired by divine prophecy, tells the messenger to relate to the king, the patient, a downright lie: tell him he will surely live, reassure him, even though prophetic inspiration imparts that the king is stricken by a fatal affliction.

On the strength of this incident in the Bible, the Talmud ruled—and subsequently this became a highly-developed point of law—that in cases where there is the slightest suspicion that by divulging the truth to the patient you may cause a mental or a physical setback, that is, may crush his hope in recovery, or create a trauma which will add to his affliction—then under no circumstances are you ethically entitled to tell the full truth to the patient. Only if you know the patient well, having established a sufficient rapport with him, and if, far from causing him a traumatic experience, this information may actually come as a relief to the patient, in that that his suffering is going to end; then, by all means, tell him. But, if it is not likely that the patient will benefit, then you should not risk aggravating his condition by telling him.

It will immediately be seen that we are here at variance in our attitude from the teachings of other faiths that tell that you must inform the patient if he is not expected to live. This approach exists notably among Catholics, for instance, who insist on telling the patient so that he can prepare himself and receive the sacraments. We do not share that attitude. We say, we would gladly sacrifice all the spiritual interests of the patient by giving priority to his physical welfare. Therefore, his physical well-being must be our first consideration, even if it is achieved at the cost of his not being able to make temporal or spiritual preparations for death.

Nor do we share the view widely held among doctors, in this country even more than in Britain—that in case of any doubt, you do tell the patient. Today this is often the general tendency. Of course, a doctor who tells a patient that he is fatally stricken cannot go wrong. If the patient dies in due course, then of course the doctor made the correct diagnosis. Should a miracle happen, and the patient survive despite the fatal diagnosis, then the doctor is an even greater doctor: he worked a miracle. We oppose this attitude, and on the strength of a strict biblical precedent going back to the passage mentioned from the Book of Kings, we would always give the physical welfare of the patient first consideration. This is the primary consideration in the whole doctor-patient relationship (and, for that matter, in the relationship between the patient and members of his family).

From this, let us proceed to some far more complex issues. These have become more acute and urgent with the opportunities we now have for artificial resuscitation or the maintenance of life functions with machinery such as respirators and heart/lung machines; as well as the enormous pressures to utilize human beings at the brink of death for, say, transplant purposes as donors. If a donor kidney, or heart, is needed, this vital organ must be taken while it is still functioning; hence the pressure to define the moment of death at the earliest possible time. Hence also, the pressure to determine at what stage we can release hospital authorities from the enormous burden imposed on their limited resources and allow artificial resuscitation or life-support systems to be stopped, and to be made available to the next patient. These modern advances raise, with increasing urgency, questions of the most acute nature not only regarding the precise definition of death, but also on the necessity of applying heroic or extraordinary methods to maintain a life that is already in its flickering stage.

In trying to deal with this whole area of the terminal stage of illness and ethical attitudes towards it, we must revert to consideration of what it is, basically, that makes Judaism *tick*. What is the underlying rationale for our whole approach? How do we apply timeless principles, which are enunciated in much earlier sources, to these highly modern situations that perplex the administration of contemporary medicine, and which increase almost daily?

What we are dealing with here is fundamentally not the definition of death, but of life. We have to define what we mean by the sanctity of life. When we regard a human being as precious and believe it is urgent to maintain life, what is the underlying criterion for the value of life? To what extent does that definition have a bearing on our right, at some point, to surrender our efforts to maintain life, or indeed to define life as having ceased and death as having supervened? Jewish law abhors the vagueness of generalities and abstractions in the same way as nature abhors a vacuum. "The sanctity of life," therefore, about which we so glibly talk, is quite an un-Jewish expression.

Hence, we would like to translate this vague notion of the sanctity of life into something much more specific—something that can be applied more immediately in legal and moral terms, in ethical as well as religious terms. Jewish law defines every human life (let me emphasize that in refering to human life, I am only dealing with innocent human life and not human life which deserves capital punishment as determined by Jewish law) as being infinite in value.

The operative term is the word "infinite." Anybody familiar with even the rudiments of mathematics knows that infinity is indivisible. No matter how many times you divide infinity, by a thousand or by a million, every fraction of infinity remains infinite. It remains exactly what you started out with. Once we define human life as being infinite in value, it follows that if 70 years of life are of infinite worth, then half of that—35 years of life, or 10 years of life, or 5 years of life, or a week of life, or an hour of life, or a split second of life—all are equally infinite in value, because infinity is indivisible.

It may quite reasonably be argued that this sounds perfectly plausible and irrefutable in terms of logic and mathematics. But why insist on defining the value of life as being infinite to the point that it is indivisible—that every fraction of life is worth as much as the totality of life?

Suppose we determine through the latest diagnostic methods, or (to take the example a step further), through prophetic inspiration, that a patient has an hour to live. Let us assume we know with certainty that this patient can only live one more hour, and that this hour will bring suffering to him and his family and be an ordeal for all involved. And then let us reason that this life, this one hour, being worse than worthless, we can cut short; causing him to die an hour earlier than he would otherwise die.

It would then follow that another patient who does not have one more hour to live, but two more hours to live, has twice that infinitesimal value, whatever it may be. Accordingly, other patients who have another week to go, or another month to live, or another 3 months or another 6 months, or another year or another 5 years or 10 years, would proportionately increase in value. The greater the expectancy of life, the greater such patients' worth, and the greater the value of their life. This, to Judaism, is utterly unacceptable, because it would undermine the very foundation of the moral order according to which we all have an equal claim to life.

The moment that you define life, or the value of life, as depending on any arbitrary criterion such as the expectancy of life (whereby someone who can still look forward to 70 years is worth more than someone who only is likely to live another 10 years, or another week, or another hour), you begin grading human beings into some who are worth more and others who are worth less. This leads directly to the Nazi doctrine that divided human beings into superiors and inferiors. Some, like the Teutonic race or the "master race," were considered worth saving at all costs. Others, like Jews and gypsies, were considered inferior, and hence not worth preserving. They could thus be shoved into the ovens by the millions.

By defining the value of human life in terms of the expectancy of life, there is taken away from all of us, from every human being, our absolute value, and a merely relative value is ascribed. Our lives would then possess a value relative to either the time we still have to live, or our state of health, or our usefulness to society, or any other arbitrary criterion. This is intolerable from a moral point of view.

Hence we say that, as deeply as we care about relieving human suffering, the one thing that we cannot do is to purchase relief of human suffering at the cost of life itself—in other words, by killing the patient. That is the one means we cannot use to bring his ordeal to an end. The moment we sacrifice a single patient because his life had become "worthless," we reduce the worth of all human lives from being absolute and inviolate to something relative, and people are graded into those who are worth more and those who are worth less. For this reason we can no more sacrifice the one hour of the patient who has only one hour to live than we can sacrifice the 70 years of life that somebody else may still anticipate.

There is no question, therefore, to Judaism, of absolute and unconditional opposition to any form of direct or active euthanasia, of deliberately hastening the end: the injection of air into the veins, the administration of any overdose of lethal drugs, or the like. Any physician deliberately causing a patient to die, under whatever conditions of debility or suffering, is regarded as committing an act of first degree murder. Nor would any account whatsoever be taken of the wishes of the patient. We are no more masters over our own lives, than we are masters over anyone else's. Just as we have no right to commit an act of murder against someone else, we have no right to murder ourselves, or to forego our absolute claim to life by giving consent to its destruction.

What is now being considered in the increasing rabbinic literature on this highly complex subject is not the administration of a killing agent to the patient (which is not tolerated under any circumstances), but the withdrawal of *artificial* means of sustaining a lingering life in order to shorten the patient's agony. There are authorities, leading rabbinic sages of our day,[1] who have ruled permissively in such cases and would allow, under carefully defined circumstances, medical aid of an artificial nature to be withdrawn from a patient in the terminal stage of a fatal condition. They would then let nature take its course.

Consider, for instance, an automobile accident case, in which the victim is admitted to a casualty ward in a hopeless condition. It is established that irreversible brain damage has occurred; but if he were put on a machine, the vital life functions could be maintained for some time, possibly indefinitely. According to liberal interpretations, we may in such circumstances withhold this life support system with a view to reducing the dying agony.

Or, to take a rather more sweeping example. Modern rabbinic authorities would hold that if a cancer patient in the terminal stage contracts pneumonia, and artificial means such as antibiotics would have to be applied in order to kill the infection, these may not be required in such a case, in as much as such treatment would serve only to prolong the dying agony. (This assumes that every single such case would be submitted to competent medical judgment in consultation with equally competent moral authorities—rabbis in the case of those who submit to Jewish law—and that each case is individually judged to comply with these careful definitions as given.)

There are, however, other authorities of equal rank[1] who are not prepared to extend such permissive rulings. They would, in general, require everything to be done that is humanly possible (including the application of artificial means) to prolong life, because of its infinite value. Therefore, a definitive ruling one way or the other cannot be indicated. The matter is still moot and very much under discussion. But those who follow the more lenient, permissive line have very good and reliable authorities on which to base their judgments.

In regard to the definition of death, as to the moment we

regard a life as having ceased, to the extent that, say, vital organs can be removed for transplant purposes—at what moment can such action be taken on the assumption that death has definitely occurred? To offer just a broad indication of the direction that Jewish thought and law takes in resolving this problem: We will certainly not accept as final and absolute the commonly held definition of "clinical" death. Clinical death means that a form of death has taken place, but certainly not a full complete death; otherwise they would not use the expression "clinical death." In other words, some biological life functions still exist; but to all intents and purposes, "clinically" speaking, the patient is regarded as dead. Generally, clinical death involves some irreversible damage to the central nerve center, more especially the brain stem.

Again, loosely speaking, irreversible brain damage is commonly identified with clinical death and this definition is now widely accepted. There is little legislation on this as yet in Western countries, but in practice this definition is widely regarded as sufficient for practical application in routine hospital procedures. Jewish law cannot accept this as absolute in defining death, and we would certainly regard any spontaneous life function still being maintained—notably respiration, (breathing) and pulsation, (heart function)—as indicating that a patient is still alive, whatever the condition of the brain. This makes it inadmissible to kill him by removing a vital organ.

Similarly, to put it in more lay terms, it would not occur to any coroner in England (called medical examiners in the US) to release a body for burial, or for that matter to let an undertaker carry out the burial, if the heart is still beating in the patient, no matter what the condition of the brain. We would regard any removal of vital organs from a patient before all spontaneous life functions had ceased as acts of killing, of homicide, indeed of murder. It is for this reason that we urge the utmost caution in operations that require the transfer of a vital organ from one person to another, from a donor to a recipient.

I will not here enter into the wider issue of transplants, especially of heart transplants, where very often of course the risk is not only to the donor, but to the recipient as well. Some years ago I had a long discussion with Dr. Christian Barnard, the pioneer of heart transplant surgery in South Africa, in this regard. I need hardly tell you that our respective moral definitions of death are not identical, and that we had some mutually provocative arguments during this most fascinating hour we spent together. So we would not only be very deeply concerned not to hasten the death of the donor, but be equally concerned with the recipient. We would want to ensure that the procedure is advanced enough and has been sufficiently tested, especially on animals, to deal with the problem of rejection. It must have passed the purely experimental stage, and allow for a reasonable anticipation of success on the part of the recipient. Were such a procedure practiced purely for research purposes, we would not endorse it.

I have sketched a few of the practical applications of those teachings that are enshrined in much earlier sources and are gradually being applied through the process of the evolution of Jewish law. This is the dynamic on the strength of which Jewish law operates. It responds to situations that demand an ethical and moral dimension in medicine—as indeed in science and technology—to exert constraints which may ultimately determine the survival of human life itself.

I need hardly remind you—living here, close to the heartland of the new space age and all it stands for, and not very far from places where the first atomic tests were carried out—of the brinkmanship that human society today experiences. For the first time since the days of Noah's flood, the survival of the human species itself may be at risk if we do not succeed in checking the enormous energies that we can now harness and then release for human destruction.

Likewise, in our drive to mechanize medicine, we may lose the human factor—that which transcends the mere mechanics of human existence. We must therefore apply checks and balances, constraints and controls that will ensure that we remain masters over our purely mechanical abilities to sustain and to resuscitate human life. Unless we succeed in that, we will reduce human beings into mere machine parts or machine tools. We will mechanize human life and deprive every human being of his uniqueness and his incomparable spirituality—his soul, as some call it, that extra feature which makes the difference between a mechanical object and a human being. It gives man the ingenuity and the insight to become a partner with God the Creator Himself, both in the generation of life and in the enrichment of life. This alone is the guarantee that we may save humanity from the disaster that lurks, and from the immeasurable threats that weigh heavily on the conscience of all charged with the destiny of the human race.

I would like to close by suggesting that we as a people have, for nearly 4,000 years, dedicated our whole national purpose, our whole national existence, to pioneering the moral law. We have, for long periods of history, been very lonely indeed. We lived in a pagan world that did not share our most basic concepts of social justice and human brotherhood under the fatherhood of God; of the moral law, and the absolute standards of the moral law. We have persevered because of our infinite dedication to this national purpose for which we were elected, and whose contribution was to be our historic assignment; it is because of this that we have survived and are here to tell the story.

We could also, as a nation, have preferred the euthanasia of a pleasant death to our election as a people with a special purpose. We could have given up our uniqueness and joined the majority, and have disappeared as so many other bigger nations disappeared. If we nonetheless determined to remain alive despite a great deal of suffering, it was because we were convinced that where there is life, there is hope. If redemption had not occurred in past generations, it would happen in some future generation: the dawn of a new era would rise upon our fortunes; we would return to our land; we would once again become a people in charge of ourselves, of our corporate destiny and responsibility, so that we might once more resume our historic assignment. We have begun to fulfill that dream by returning to our national purpose—especially in magnificent institutions such as Cedars-Sinai Medical Center dedicated to healing—in a Jewish context and in a Jewish dimension. We longed for a return to enriching the human experience by being once more moral pioneers, particularly in a sphere in which we have contributed, both as doctors and as moral specialists, so much to the health of mankind and to the advancement of medicine. The hope is that we will eventually play a renewed role in restoring that sanity, mental and physical, in human relations, which alone will fulfill our vision of the brotherhood of man under the fatherhood of God.

NOTE

1. For some of these conflicting opinions among contemporary Halachists, see Immanuel Jakobovits, *Jewish Medical Ethics,* new edition, 1975, p. 276.

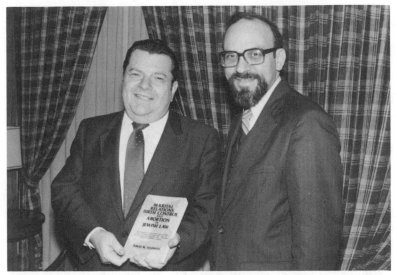

Rabbi David M. Feldman, D.H.L. and Rabbi Levi Meier, Ph.D.

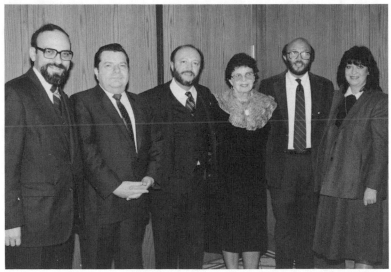

Rabbi Levi Meier, Ph.D.; Rabbi David M. Feldman, D.H.L.; Allen Salick, M.D.; Mrs. Blanche Salick; Bernard Salick, M.D.; and Renee Salick, Ph.D.

Bill Watson

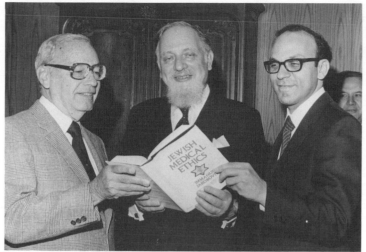

*Robert L. Spencer, Chairman of the Board, Cedars-Sinai Medical Center;
Sir Immanuel Jakobovits, Ph.D.; and Rabbi Levi Meier, Ph.D.*

Bill Watson

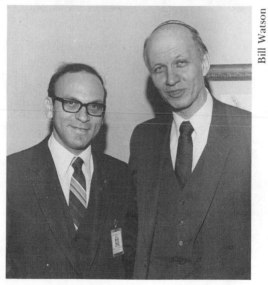

Rabbi Levi Meier, Ph.D. and Rabbi Irving Greenberg, Ph.D.

97

Bill Watson

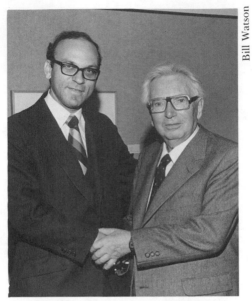

Rabbi Levi Meier, Ph.D. and Viktor E. Frankl, M.D., Ph.D.

Owen

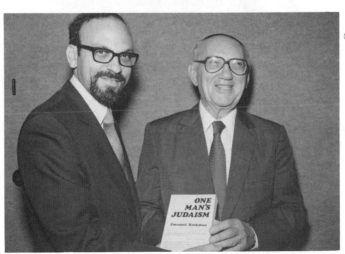

Rabbi Levi Meier, Ph.D. and Rabbi Emanuel Rackman, Ph.D.

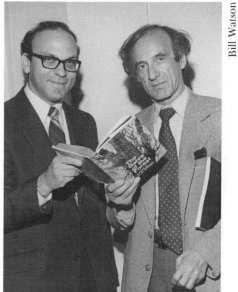

Bill Watson

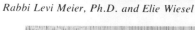

Rabbi Levi Meier, Ph.D. and Elie Wiesel

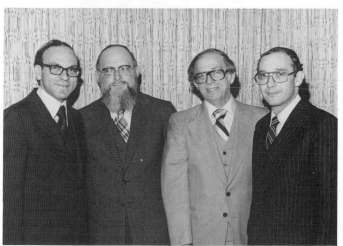

Bill Watson

Rabbi Levi Meier,Ph.D.; Rabbi J. David Bleich, Ph.D.;
Rabbi Paul Dubin and Fred Rosner, M.D.

Part II

7

A Singular Patient

Elie Wiesel

I must tell you that I agreed to come here because I like the idea of having physicians, surgeons, psychiatrists engage in an educational process; and I shall tell you why. In our times, there is usually a total dichotomy between education and medicine, between the humanities and medicine, between medicine and all the—so to speak—literary activities. Unfortunately, we are told, the moment a person goes to medical school, he or she will stop reading books. So I felt that maybe this would be the opportunity for me to tell you about all the books you have not read.

At the same time, I must tell you I feel a special relationship to doctors, first because they helped me so often; I needed them so often. Also because in our tradition the doctor occupies an ambivalent place. On the one hand, God seems to be jealous of the doctor, because He says, "Adoshem rofeh cholim"—*He* cures the patient. It may be an act of jealousy. Otherwise, why wouldn't He say, "I am the one who writes books?" He does not take this title; He wants the MD. On the other hand, we have in the Talmud the strange passage which states, *"Tov shebarof'im le-Gehinom"*—the best of the doctors go to hell. And my interpretation of this is, *"Tov shebarof'im,"* the best of the doctors are *needed* in *Gehinom*.

I thought about this on two occasions. In 1979 or 1980, I went to the Cambodian border to see what was happening there immediately after Pol Pot and his killers revealed themselves for what they were. There I met Jewish doctors, some from Israel and some from the United States. They were the first to come, and I cannot tell you how proud I felt, proud that the very first to come and help those Cambodian refugees, men, women and children, were Jewish doctors. But then, I thought of another period, a strange period too. In 1945, when most of you were still in high school, the war ended and the DP camps began their legendary existence. I was told by friends liberated from Bergen-Belsen that although there was an epidemic in 1945, not a single doctor left his or her practice to come and take care of the refugees there. That hurt. I don't know why. During the war, of course, the World War II was going on. But afterwards, what held them back?

What space is there between the words "Holocaust" and "patient"? The great Hasidic master, Levi-Yitzhak of Berditchev, used to say that when the Messiah will come, we will understand not only the words in the Torah but also the space that separates the words. Apparently, he was suggesting that between words there is something else, and sometimes what is there has more meaning than the words themselves. What is the space separating "Holocaust" from "patient"?

After the war, I was in Paris studying philosophy. In France, if you study philosophy, you must also take a secondary subject, and I took psychiatry. So I spent 2 years studying and working in an institution. I didn't know why then, but now I think I do. From the very beginning we had a feeling that something had happened in those years that was so far beyond understanding that it could only be thought of as a mental aberration on a cosmic scale. Therefore, I wanted to understand what had happened then by using the tools, the vehicles, and the vast resources of medicine or psychiatry. Not through philosophy: philosophy had failed, and therefore I failed to even come close to the problem by applying philosophical terms. Literature was better, and that is why I love literature. I came to philosophy because of the questions, and I left it because of the answers. There are no answers. Everything is a question. So I studied and I wanted to see what went wrong.

Surely, some of you know, those of you who were there, that whenever a person arrived in that strange kingdom, he or she was struck by its vastness, its infinite dimension. Suddenly you dicovered that the infinite exists, and it is there before you. The infinite number of victims. The infinite expanse of barbed wire. Suddenly the infinite was there. And you realized that evil had more power than good, because one rifle was stronger than a thousand poems written by a thousand poets. What we wanted then to understand, as the testimony of every survivor shows, was the meaning of it all. It had to have a meaning. What did it all mean? We felt, somehow we felt, that an experiment had been undertaken there. These were not simply a bunch of killers who began killing. They had an idea behind it. Theirs was a kind of laboratory from the perspective of history and metaphysics. They wanted to prove something; to create a new man. Maybe to start history all over again. You know they were obsessed with that.

Throughout the war, Himmler, the head of the Gestapo and the SS, was fascinated with the theories of the Aryan society and he sought to find a kind of primary, primordial man. Throughout the war, he sent delegations of so-called scientists to India where the Aryan races began, to the Himalayas, to Tibet. I am convinced they had an idea there. They wanted to prove, to uncover, to establish something new, and Himmler wanted to understand its meaning. He didn't find any point of reference.

As a child, since I was still a child in those times, my point of reference was the Inquisition. When I saw the flames, I thought of the Inquisition and its flames. But I needed that point; I needed a point of return. I needed to know that there was an event like it before, and therefore the meaning from the past could apply to the present. Except I was wrong. There was no event like it, and I think there never will be.

What was it? Was it a trauma; was it an aberration of history? Or, on the contrary, was it a culmination of history? On the one hand, you cannot escape the notion that it was set in history. It happened in a certain place; it was done by a certain group of people to a group of people, using certain methods, invoking certain ideas. The whole structure proved to be functional. The system worked. That is what was so strange. You came into that system and you saw the killer kill, the watchmen watch, and you saw the prisoners run around. It worked. What made it work? What kind of madness was it?

This trauma actually should change any person who comes in touch with it. If you, as physicians, surgeons, or teachers come in touch with that period, it must change your life because you realize suddenly that whatever you do today must be judged and measured by those times, against the background of those flames. You cannot avoid it. Once you become aware, whatever you do takes on a different meaning. Somehow the futilities of daily existence seem more futile, because you realize that every minute is a minute of grace, and you had better do something with it. Maybe if you were spared, as we were spared, there was no meaning to it, but we must confer a meaning on it now—retroactively.

If you think in those terms, then the teacher teaches differently, the healer heals differently, and the patient suffers differently.

What Rabbi Meier[1] said about the patient interested me very much. Why do they talk to you about that period? Is it because you are a rabbi, and therefore, as a rabbi you are used to suffering? Or is it simply because they realize that you know things that they don't, and they want to share with you; or is it because they, too, in their moments of stress, needed a vantage point?

I get many letters from readers, mainly children. I get around a hundred letters from children a month and I answer every single one of them. They usually write to me after reading *Night* or *Dawn*. I wish they would read other books I have written. Actually, I have written very few on the Holocaust. Of my 21, only four deal with that period. But the children read those, and of course it is rewarding and heartbreaking at the same time. Those who write to me and who are not children are patients: mainly cancer patients, or their parents or their wives or husbands or their brethren. Somehow they feel that the only person who could understand the cancer patient, who could talk to a cancer patient, is someone who went through that period, and maybe it is true. Because during that time we witnessed the extreme, we evolved beyond the extreme of suffering. Therefore the cancer patient wants to know how you dealt with it. How did you live? How did you accept life? But the parents of the cancer patient also want to know how you accepted life afterwards? How did you adjust? So maybe you know. I am sure you know, because you are in touch with suffering. Therefore, I respect you.

After the war, our educators were wrong. I was young, I came to Paris, and only much later, some 20 or 30 years later, I found out that they were in awe of our presence, because we children knew so much more than they did. We knew so much more about life and death and truth and language and history—everything. We *knew* everything. They thought that they were brought in by the French government or by Jewish organizations to help us adjust to life. They were wrong: our problem was how to adjust to death. Death during the war was an everyday phenomenon, a casual incident—it was nothing. You were used to it. You were used to sleeping with corpses, and getting up and seeing more corpses around you. Death was no longer a scandal in Creation. It was part of, if not a dominant motif, in Creation. After the war, we had to learn new attitudes towards death; we had to learn to face death with new respect, awe, and fear. In other words, we had to learn how to live after our encounter with death, after death, and that is why the cancer patients and their parents want to know from us the "after." How do you do it?

Normally, we survivors should be abnormal. Anyone who was alive during that trauma must be singed by its flames. And, therefore, it would be normal for any one of us not to be normal. But let me tell you the answer of a very great teacher, HaRav Kahaneman, the *Rosh Yeshiva* (rabbi) from Ponevez Yeshiva, who took his entire yeshiva during the war through China and Japan, bringing them to America, and managing thereby to save all of his *talmidim* (students). When he was asked afterwards where he got all the strength and energy to work for his yeshiva, he said, "I will tell you: the war made us all insane—mad. Some people used their madness to make money; others to get honor. I use my madness to teach." That is the most creative way I have ever heard to describe the survivor's madness and its metamorphosis into something therapeutic. You don't ignore it; it is there. How can you possibly ignore it? But once you confront it head on and you know its intensity, its bite, you try to do something with it. Not something *against* mankind, but something *for* mankind.

As a Jew, of course, mankind appears to me through the fate of the Jewish people and Jewish history. I don't have to apologize for it. I am what I am. I accept my heritage as a privilege and therefore whatever I do, I do with that sense of privilege. If I went to Cambodia, I went there as a Jew, because as a Jew, I had to be there. If I am concerned about every tragedy that happens today, it is the Jew in me who is concerned. If now, for instance, I am so terribly scared about the nuclear menace, it is the Jew in me who is scared—because I already know that the impossible is not really impossible. Once you have the words, the content of the words will come to pass. Once we have invented the idea that the planet can destroy itself simply because of an error or because of an idiot somewhere in Libya or in Uganda, then I don't see how the planet can be saved unless tremendous awareness takes place.

May I tell you one more thought? I confide it with a genuine sense of respect for what you are doing. What hurt us during the war was not only the realization that humanity can be so easily dehumanized—I am not speaking of the dehumanization of the victim which was done and perfected by the killer. I am speaking of the dehumanization of the killer. What hurt was that there were people—and to this day I don't understand it—there were intelligent people in the Einsatz commandos. The Einsatz commandos were the worst, because they had followed the front and systematically killed Jews from the very moment that war had begun in Poland—hence even before the Final Solution had emerged from the Wansee Conference.

Babi Yar occurred 10 days after the Germans invaded Kiev. That happened between Rosh Hashana and Yom Kippur: day after day, 10,000 men, women, and children would come to the pit, undress, and—I must interrupt to relate two things: Babi Yar is not far away. It is not, as Gertrude Stein said, "there"; it is not "there." Babi Yar was *here,* meaning it was part of Kiev, not outside Kiev. When I visited there for the first time, I was shocked. I thought Babi Yar must be a forest somewhere, hidden away. It is part of Kiev, 10 minutes away from the hotel where we stayed. The people of Kiev heard the machine guns—and the Germans did not kill at night. They killed during the day. I asked the Russians about this when I was there because I could not understand. They were angry. I asked what happened to them; why didn't they open their doors?

Do you know that when a few people, a very few, managed to crawl out from under the corpses, naked, they would run away at night because the Germans stopped killing at night? They would run to a nearby hut a few meters or kilometers away, and they would not be allowed in. Peasants would say, "Jew, go back to the grave." One Jew was clever—he was a yeshiva *bocher* (student): he came to a farm, knocked at the door; the peasant woman opened it and then sent him away. But he knocked again; he had a marvelous inspiration. When she opened the door this time, ready to send him away again, he said—standing there naked— "Don't send me away, I am your Lord Jesus Christ." She was a peasant woman; she believed him. He was covered with blood, with stigmata. So she hid him for three days, and then he ran into the forest to join the partisans. Why didn't the Russians allow Jews inside their huts?

But worst of all, those who did the killing were not cheap mafia murderers. Most of them were educated people. To this day, I take my head in my hands and I wonder how it could have been. Most of them had degrees, college degrees, doctorates. It was not an easy thing then to get a doctorate in Germany—a PhD in philosophy, in jurisprudence, in theology, in the arts. Opera singers were among the killers. These people did the direct killing—not even handling corpses with gloves as they did afterwards in Auschwitz— they did the brutal killing. How can one be a college graduate with a PhD in divinity, appreciate the beauty of a sonnet, admire a painting by Goya, and kill? How is it that culture did not provide a shield? I have no answer. But I know it happened.

What do I learn from this? I learn that culture without conscience is not culture. Science without culture will turn against man. Therefore, together with you, I would like to urge all the universities with which we are affiliated, to impose courses in the humanities for doctors, engineers, and scientists. We must know—they must know—what life is all about. I do not think that *anyone* could do what the killers did. I do not believe in analogies. That event is beyond analogy, but I believe in its implications. That Jewish tragedy had universal implications, and therefore we must learn and go on learning and go on studying all about it. What made the killers inhuman? I don't know. Was it their numbness? Was it what they were taught for so many centuries— that the Jew is not a human being? That the Jew is subhuman? Was it because they, too, remembered the Inquisition? I have seen a print of a medieval painting showing the way they burned the Jews at the stake during the Inquisition: the wood and the fire, the faces of the victims. You can see the drawing in any encyclopedia. What is astonishing is that it is exactly the same method used by the Germans, by the killers in Treblinka and in Majdanek. Did they, too, inherit something from their collective memory: how to do it?

I have recently read a book about the massacres in White Russia and Lithuania. I read everything. Strangely enough, those of us who were there read more than those who were not there. I read everything; I want to know as much as I can. I want to enlarge the area of my understanding. I always hope that maybe I will find something new, that then I will understand the meaning of it all. So I read, and read, and read. A few months ago, I read *The Black Book,* eyewitness accounts collected by Ilya Ehrenburg and another Jewish writer in Russia named Vasili Grossman. You read it, and at one point, you must stop—you cannot continue: first-person accounts about everything, about the Ukraine and Rumania and Babi Yar and Minsk. I do not know the answers to how and why and what, but the questions are there. And I shall leave you with one image, an account of a Jewish woman and her family who were hiding in a cave somewhere in Kiev. They decided to run away and go the countryside. The mother and her two children tried to sneak out during the day and go to some village. They were stopped by a military unit. You read the story, which I can repeat only with difficulty, and you have nightmares. This is almost a direct quote: The military men caught that family and began torturing them, tormenting them, ridiculing them, laughing at them, laughing. Then one of them took a child, one of the two, and beheaded the child. Then he took the second child and beheaded the second child. And then, says the witness, the mother, insane with grief, took her two dead children and she began to dance with them. The killers went on laughing and she went on dancing. I don't know what she saw. I know that unless we try to visualize her, then the killers will be going on with their laughter.

But suffering and agony are not the whole story. *Resistance* is part of it. There was no ghetto without a movement of resistance. There were resistance movements even in the death camps. Which means that no other nation, no other people in occupied Europe showed such a spirit of resistance as the Jewish people. The first civil uprising was not Paris, not Warsaw, but the Warsaw ghetto. That is true of Bialystock, of Vilna, of everyplace. Factually, the answer is that they did resist, but it is almost irrelevant because that is not the problem. The problem lies beyond that. We are dealing with something that we cannot even articulate. What happened to humanity? How is it possible that human beings can do such things to other human beings? To children? One million—more—were children. How many hours do you doctors spend in a day, every day, trying to save one life, of one child? And there you had human beings killing children in the name of some demented ideal, which to the killers was reasonable and rational, even lofty.

Now let us consider the question from a different angle. One million were children. And we want children to organize resistance? Babies? And at least one million were old people. You want them to organize? You want the rabbis to launch military campaigns? You want the old hasidim (pious people) to work out strategic attacks? Or the sick? How many *were* there who could have organized resistance movements? Many of them were old women. Where would they have gotten a tradition of resistance? The miracle is that they *did* resist, and that is to me the greatest source of astonishment.

When the Warsaw ghetto rose up in arms, the high command, the entire high command, were in their teens. If you took all of them together, their ages did not add up to 120 years. The oldest was Mordechai Anielewicz, who, since Bar Kochba, had nobody to refer to as a vantage point. Others were youngsters: youngsters who one day decided to take Jewish history on their shoulders and say, we are doing something that 18 centuries of Jews didn't do.

Every occupied nation had a parallel home organization in London or Moscow or Washington, that gave them arms, sent messengers, instructors, and kept up the liaison, to enable them to fight. The only group that received *no* help from anyone was the Jewish underground. With what could they fight? When they received the first weapon, the first gun, which they bought with gold, and that is not a metaphor—it was with *gold*—they wept. And we have descriptions, because we had chronicles in every camp and in every ghetto, of how they learned to fire a gun. With a few guns, they decided to defy what was then the mightiest army in Europe. Remember, this was 1943. True, it was after Stalingrad, but a year and a half before Normandy. And they decided to brave the German army. Do you know that it took the Germans longer to conquer the Warsaw ghetto than to occupy France? This is what I don't understand. Where did the Jews get the courage, the faith, let alone the knowledge that was required for anyone to go and fight?

There were other forms of resistance: spiritual resistance. There were schools in every ghetto. There were artistic enterprises in every camp. Adorno, a German philosopher, said there is no poetry after Auschwitz. He is right, though not entirely. There was poetry *inside* Auschwitz, where Jews studied, learned, tried to help one another so that they were not dehumanized. That is something which will always resonate in me as long as I live.

Naturally, I referred to Jewish victims. What about the others? There was a difference. Only a Jew was condemned for his or her being. *Being* became a crime. Being Jewish was cause enough to be sentenced to death. Children were playing in the gardens of my town, or in Budapest, in Lodz, or in Debrecen, anywhere; they were already dead but they didn't know it. Because in Berlin the killers had already decided that these children were dead. Why? Because they were Jewish. Not even the gypsies were treated with such a ruthless, brutal attitude. Furthermore, and this is very serious; I think you—who asked a question about Jewish violence—are too harsh on yourself. In our tradition, a killer is a person who killed, but only a person who has already killed, not a potential killer. Cain was a killer after he killed Abel, but not before. And until a person is a killer, a person really need not see himself or herself as a potential killer. That is, none of our Sages has asked us to go that far with self-identification. It is difficult enough for you to imagine yourself a victim: therefore, stay there. Don't go further.

It is enough. Who am I to tell you all this? I occupy no function. I am really a person alone, alone with my writings and with my students.

My attitude towards Israel? Even there we should not be too harsh. Demanding, yes: we should expect almost the impossible from ourselves, but, at the same time, we must not judge a people that is 3,500 years old—not by single episodes. It is my conviction, my *Ani Maamin* (belief), that one day—and the day may be soon—there will be a new relationship, maybe even a nonagression pact leading to peace, between the Palestinian people and Israel. I do not know how, because I am not a politician. But when I go to Israel, and I go there at least once a year, I see what the conflict is doing to Israel. The young people, the children, the young soldiers who have to serve in the occupied territories—they don't like it. I remember; after the Six-Day war, Yitzhak Rabin, the army's Commander-in-Chief, and his senior staff had difficulties finding officers to serve as military governors in the newly occupied territories. Now, if you study—and I am sure you have studied—history, there is nothing as pleasant for an officer as being a military governor, because he is powerful, he can have everything. He is treated like a king. He has the powers of a king.

Not in Israel. They could not find candidates for military governors. No one wanted the job. They didn't want to rule over other people. In the Jewish tradition, victory is always victory over ourselves, not over the enemy: never. It is always an inward, a moral act that we demand from ourselves, but which we don't ever expect from others. So therefore, I am convinced that never, never will Jewish soldiers ever be compared to the Germans' accomplices, let alone to the Germans themselves. I don't know how they could be. All I can convey to you is my hope that by your listening and sharing, by your accepting, you become the repository of stories you cannot even imagine. By accepting the remembrance of things that you have not lived through, by becoming their witnesses, you can accept yourself. Those who come to you, need you. But I think that ultimately you will realize that you need them—the survivors—as much as, if not more than, they need you, because they possess something which is now, and will remain, the very center, the core of what constitutes the texture and the fabric of Jewish sensitivity, if not of Jewish memory.

NOTE

1. During my pastoral rounds as chaplain, the majority of patients mention the Holocaust and its effects on them within the first 10 to 15 minutes of my conversation with them. The patients' comments usually reflect a few of the following typological responses: A patient may say, this is my second spouse; my first wife or husband and children died in the camps. Or they may say; yesterday I was in the camps and today I need major surgery, and nothing has happened during the last 40 years. Or; if I survived the Holocaust I'll survive this surgery as well. Or, is this what I survived for?

8

The Meaning of
Suffering*

Viktor E. Frankl, M.D., Ph.D.

There are three main avenues on which one arrives at meaning in life. The first is by creating a work or by doing a deed. The second is by experiencing something or encountering someone; in other words, meaning can be found not only in work but also in love. Edith Weisskopf-Joelson observed in this context that the logotherapeutic "notion that experiencing can be as valuable as achieving is therapeutic because it compensates for our one-sided emphasis on the external world of achievement at the expense of the internal world of experience."[1]

Most important, however, is the third avenue to meaning in life: even the helpless victim of a hopeless situation, facing a fate he cannot change, may rise above himself, may grow beyond himself, and by so doing change himself. He may turn a personal tragedy into a triumph. Again, it was Edith Weisskopf-Joelson who once expressed the hope that lo-

*Reprinted from *Man's Search for Meaning* by permission of Beacon Press. Copyright © 1984 by Viktor Frankl.

gotherapy "may help counteract certain unhealthy trends in the present-day culture of the United States, where the incurable sufferer is given very little opportunity to be proud of his suffering and to consider it ennobling rather than degrading" so that "he is not only unhappy, but also ashamed of being unhappy."

For a quarter of a century I ran the neurological department of a general hospital and bore witness to my patients' capacity to turn their predicaments into human achievements. In addition to such practical experience, empirical evidence is also available which supports the possibility that one may find meaning in suffering. Researchers at the Yale University School of Medicine "have been impressed by the number of prisoners of war of the Vietnam war who explicitly claimed that although their captivity was extraordinarily stressful—filled with torture, disease, malnutrition, and solitary confinement—they nevertheless . . . benefited from the captivity experience, seeing it as a growth experience."[2]

But the most powerful arguments in favor of "a tragic optimism" are those which in Latin are called *argumenta ad hominem*. Jerry Long, to cite an example, is a living testimony to "the defiant power of the human spirit," as it is called in logotherapy.[3] To quote the *Texarkana Gazette,* "Jerry Long has been paralyzed from his neck down since a diving accident which rendered him a quadriplegic 3 years ago. He was 17 when the accident occurred. Today Long can use his mouth stick to type. He 'attends' two courses at Community College via a special telephone. The intercom allows Long to both hear and participate in class discussions. He also occupies his time by reading, watching television and writing." And in a letter I received from him, he writes: "I view my life as being abundant with meaning and purpose. The attitude that I adopted on that fateful day has become my personal credo for life: I broke my neck, it didn't break me. I am currently enrolled in my first psychology course in college. I believe that my handicap will only enhance my ability to help others. I know that without the suffering, the growth that I have achieved would have been impossible.''

Is this to say that suffering is indispensable to the discovery of meaning? In no way. I only insist that meaning is available in spite of—nay, even through—suffering, provided that the suffering is unavoidable. If it is avoidable, the meaningful thing to do is to remove its cause, for unnecessary suffering is masochistic rather than heroic. If, on the other hand, one cannot change a situation that causes his suffering, he can still choose his attitude.[4] Long had not been chosen to break his neck, but he did decide not to let himself be broken by what had happened to him.

As we see, the priority stays with creatively changing the situation that causes us to suffer. But the superiority goes to the "know-how to suffer," if need be. And there is empirical evidence that—literally—the "man in the street" is of the same opinion. Austrian public-opinion pollsters recently reported that those held in highest esteem by most of the people interviewed are neither the great artists nor the great scientists, neither the great statesmen nor the great sports figures, but those who master a hard lot with their heads held high.

In turning to the second aspect of the tragic triad, namely guilt, I would like to depart from a theological concept that has always been fascinating to me. I refer to what is called *mysterium iniquitatis,* meaning, as I see it, that a crime in the final analysis remains inexplicable inasmuch as it cannot be fully traced back to biological, psychological, and/or sociological factors. Totally explaining one's crime would be tantamount to explaining away his or her guilt and to seeing in him or her not a free and responsible human being but a machine to be repaired. Even criminals themselves abhor this treatment and prefer to be held responsible for their deeds. From a convict serving his sentence in an Illinois penitentiary I received a letter in which he deplored that "the criminal never has a chance to explain himself. He is offered a variety of excuses to choose from. Society is blamed and in many instances the blame is put on the victim." Furthermore, when I addressed the prisoners in San Quentin, I told them that "you are human beings like me, and as such you were free to commit a crime, to become guilty. Now, however, you are responsible for overcoming guilt by rising above it, by growing beyond yourselves, by changing for the better." They felt understood.[5] And from Frank E. W., an ex-prisoner, I received a note which stated that he had "started a logotherapy group for ex-felons. We are 27 strong and the newer ones are staying out of prison through the peer strength of those of us from the original group. Only one returned—and he is now free."[6]

As for the concept of collective guilt, I personally think that it is totally unjustified to hold one person responsible for the behavior of another person or a collective of persons. Since the end of World War II, I have not become weary of publicly arguing against the collective guilt concept.[7] Sometimes, however, it takes a lot of didactic tricks to detach people from their superstitions. An American woman once confronted me with the reproach, "How can you still write some of your books in German, Adolf Hitler's language?" In response, I asked her if she had knives in her kitchen and when she answered that she did, I acted dismayed and shocked, exclaiming, "How can you still use knives after so many killers have used them to stab and murder their victims?" She stopped objecting to my writing books in German.

The third aspect of the tragic triad concerns death. But it concerns life as well, for at any time each of the moments of which life consists is dying, and that moment will never recur. And yet is not this transitoriness a reminder that challenges us to make the best possible use of each moment of our lives? It certainly is, and hence my imperative: *Live as if you were living for the second time and had acted as wrongly the first time as you are about to act now.*

In fact, the opportunities to act properly, the potentialities to fulfill a meaning, are affected by the irreversibility of our lives. But also the potentialities alone are so affected. For as soon as we have used an opportunity and have actualized a potential meaning, we have done so once and for all. We have rescued it into the past wherein it has been safely delivered and deposited. In the past, nothing is irretrievably lost, but rather, on the contrary, everything is irrevocably stored and treasured. To be sure, people tend to see only the stubble fields of transitoriness but overlook and forget the full granaries of the past into which they have brought the harvest of their lives: the deeds done, the loves loved, and last but not least, the sufferings they have gone through with courage and dignity.

From this one may see that there is no reason to pity old people. Instead, young people should envy them. It is true that the old have no opportunities, no possibilities in the future. But they have more than that. Instead of possibilities in the future, they have realities in the past—the potentialities they have actualized, the meanings they have fulfilled, the values they have realized—and nothing and nobody can ever remove these assets from the past.

In view of the possibility of finding meaning in suffering, life's meaning is an unconditional one, at least potentially. That unconditional meaning, however, is paralleled by the unconditional value of each and every person. It is that which warrants the indelible quality of the dignity of man. Just as life remains potentially meaningful under any conditions, even those which are most miserable, so too does the value of each and every person stay with him or her, and it does so because it is based on the values that he or she has realized in the past, and is not contingent on the usefulness that he or she may or may not retain in the present.

More specifically, this usefulness is usually defined in terms of functioning for the benefit of society. But today's society is characterized by achievement orientation, and consequently it adores people who are successful and happy and, in particular, it adores the young. It virtually ignores the value of all those who are otherwise, and in so doing blurs the decisive difference between being valuable in the sense of dignity and being valuable in the sense of usefulness. If one is not cognizant of this difference and holds that an individual's value stems only from his present usefulness, then, believe me, one owes it only to personal inconsistency not to plead for euthanasia along the lines of Hitler's program, that is to say, "mercy" killing of all those who have lost their social usefulness, be it because of old age, incurable illness, mental deterioration, or whatever handicap they may suffer.

NOTES

1. The place of Logotherapy in the world today, *The International Forum for Logotherapy*, 1980 *1,* (3), 3-7.
2. Sledge, W. H., Boydstun J. A. & Rabe, A. J. Self-concept changes related to war captivity, *Archives of General Psychiatry,* 1980, *37,* 430-443.
3. "The Defiant Power of the Human Spirit" was in fact the title of a paper presented by Long at the Third World Congress of Logotherapy in June 1983.
4. I won't forget an interview I once heard on Austrian TV, given by a Polish cardiologist who, during World War II, had helped organize the Warsaw ghetto upheaval. "What a heroic deed," exclaimed the reporter. "Listen," calmly replied the doctor, "to take a gun and shoot is no great thing; but if the SS leads you to a gas chamber or to a mass grave to execute you on

the spot, and you can't do anything about it—except for going your way with dignity—you see, this is what I would call heroism." Attitudinal heroism, so to speak.

5. See also Fabry, Joseph B. *The pursuit of meaning.* New York: Harper & Row, 1980.

6. Cf. Frankl, Viktor E. *The unheard cry for meaning.* New York: Simon & Schuster, 1978, pp. 42-43.

7. See also Frankl, Viktor E. *Psychotherapy and existentialism.* New York: Simon & Schuster, 1967.

9

Toward a
Covenantal Ethic
of Medicine

Rabbi Irving Greenberg, Ph.D.

We are living in an extraordinary age of medicine, an age in which medicine (as indeed, all of human civilization) is engaged in the process of taking power—to break the overwhelming dominance of biology and nature in shaping human history. Throughout history, the fate of most human beings, in terms of personal health as well as of culture and economic and political state, has been set by the act of birth and by the given conditions of life. For most of human history, life was nasty, brutish, and short. In this age, human beings are attempting to take control of their own destiny. Nowhere is this more dramatically demonstrated than in the extraordinary explosion of power within medicine, which now begins to tackle the issues of DNA and genetic engineering and the most fundamental structures that control life itself. At such a time, it is worth looking beyond the details—to the fundamental concept of how power is directed and controlled, particularly in the medical area.

One caveat: the central religious issues involve the question of how one controls power. The tradition itself is emerging from a period of relative powerlessness and is not always psychologically or Halakhically prepared to deal with questions of power. Therefore, there must be a two-way dialogue in which the tradition has a great deal to learn from medicine, as well as medicine from the tradition.

I

In the Talmud, there is a discussion: What is *the* fundamental principle of Judaism? One answer, given by Rabbi Akiva, is that "You shall love your neighbor as yourself" is the fundamental principle from which the whole Torah is derived. His colleague Ben Azzai suggests that the fundamental principle of Judaism, and of Jewish ethics, is that the human being is created in the image of God. In the words of Genesis, "And the Lord God created the human in God's image, in the image of God, God created them, man and woman, God created them" (Genesis 1:26). This fundamental conception of the person being in the image of God is at the heart of the entire Jewish value system.

What does it mean that a human being is made in the image of God? The Talmud defines this in three ways, primarily; I will add a fourth. Firstly, human images have finite values; an image of God has infinite value. A green piece of paper with a picture of George Washington and the signature of the Treasurer of the United States is worth a dollar. A divine image has unlimited value. Therefore, the Talmud says: if you save one life, it is like saving an entire world (Sanhedrin 37A) (infinity times one is equal to infinity times billions). Secondly, there is no preferred image of God; that is to say, all images are equal. Contrary to popular rumor, God is not a Caucasian male with a white beard. Thirdly, each divine image is unique. Human images are repetitive. If a doctor reads a brain scan in which he detects abnormalities, this reflects a problem. But when it comes to human beings, i.e., images of God, "if you've seen one, you haven't seen them all."

There is a fourth dimension to being in the image of God. Normally, Judaism rejects images of God; the Second Commandment prohibits making them. What makes the human image of God different—a *positive* image? The Jewish tradition prohibits a *fixed* image of God. Making a statue of God, or taking money, or any other object and making it into the absolute—that is prohibited. Making a fixed image of God is forbidden; it is idolatry. What is unique about the human image is that it is not fixed; it is developing. Just as God is beyond description or capture in one picture or object, so is the human. For the human is unfinished, in the process of becoming; the human image of God is developing. The human divine image is becoming more and more like God, says the tradition. In humans, life is moving from the biologically fixed, (something which can be captured and exhausted), toward the psychically free. As doctors are most aware, biology is overwhelmingly determinative in human life. The congruence of DNA in the highest apes and in the humans is something like 99 percent. But the 1 percent of noncongruence is, if you will, the cutting edge of that movement from the biological to the psychic. Judaism stresses that the process of human development is a process of becoming more psychically free, more able to assert mastery and control.

Judaism makes another fundamental claim. This process of steady expansion of life, of perfection and development of life's capacity, the movement of life from pure determinism toward greater freedom, greater complexity, greater richness and greater control and consciousness, is structured into reality. To put it in theological terms, life is nurtured in the ground of God, the source of life and energy and goodness. God is moving the process toward life and perfection and toward consciousness and control.

The ultimate Jewish claim is that eventually the world itself will be restructured to support and to respect this dimension of the human being existing in the image of God. In the Messianic age there will be peace and social justice; and an infrastructure of existence rich enough to support the fullness of human dignity so that all humans will truly be treated like—and be—in the image of God. When this process reaches its final climax, life itself will be perfected—to the point of overcoming death. If you believe that, you will believe anything; but that is the fundamental Jewish claim.

What is the Jewish role in the perfection process? Judaism is a commitment: what the tradition calls a covenant. Judaism is a covenant of perfection in which the Jewish people (either as volunteers or as Chosen People, depending on interpretation) are to teach the world that perfection is the end goal. The Jewish people's mission is to teach the world not to settle for the present structure of reality, which is characterized not by the triumph of life but by sudden sickness and death, by oppression, inequity, and injustice. Judaism seeks to inject dissatisfaction into the bloodstream of humanity by teaching the world that present reality is not acceptable; it is to be corrected and redeemed. Secondly, the Jewish community, as a community, is to show people how to move toward the final perfection. After all, it is easy to talk about perfection, but how does one get there? How does one improve over the present reality without making things worse? The living community is a model of how to go about this. Last, but not least, the Jewish community is to work alongside humanity to achieve this perfection, because no one group can achieve it alone.

II

Judaism teaches that there is a covenant between God and humanity, and not just with the Jewish people. The human role in this covenant is to perfect the world which was brought into being by God: *"Le-taken olam BemalKut Shaddai*—to perfect the world with the kingdom of God." To perfect the world means that the human is called upon not to accept the world as it is, but to improve it and to complete it; not to accept the present status quo of life and death, but to change the balance of power toward life, and toward the triumph of life.

In the Book of Genesis, the first commandment to the newly created human is to rule over the earth, to shape it, to conquer it, to master it (Genesis 1:28). There is a striking contrast between Jewish culture and Eastern religion. Eastern religions contain powerful truths and insights and affirm passivity toward the world. Judaism says *not* to accept the world as it is; to *transform* it is the human calling and responsibility. The human responsibility is to fill the world with life. Since human life is in the image of God, it is a *mitzvah* to create more life, to perfect it, to move it toward this state of equality and uniqueness and infinite value. The rabbis follow this commandment (Genesis 1:28) with further instruction: *La-shevet,* the commandment to settle and civilize the world. The world as it is now is not fully civilized; it has deserts, empty spaces, all types of voids. Humans are called upon to fill those vacuums with life, and move life itself toward perfection. Therefore, the rabbis considered redemption the fundamental *human* claim and obligation, not just a Jewish responsibility. The Jews are a kind of pioneering vanguard, a model; Judaism is essentially an attempt to articulate and to develop a consciousness which the whole world is meant to achieve.

The rabbis interpreted the great symbol of ritual circumcision in this way. Take the human body given to us, affirm it; but at the same time, perfect it. The removal of the foreskin is a symbol that one does not simply accept the biological given. Rather, the human task is to perfect the body, complete it, and remove whatever imperfections it has. As the rabbis understood circumcision, it was the command to improve on biology.

How far can one push this perfection? The answer is that humans are commanded to become more and more the image of God; that is to say, more and more like God. Thus the ultimate human calling is to become as much like God as is possible. The final result would be that every possibility of life would be developed, and life would decisively triumph over death. God is pure life, containing no death. Hence the ultimate achievement of being in the divine image would be pure life and the absolute triumph of life. Isaiah in his description of the Messianic period uses that language specifically: *"belah ha-mavet la-netzach"*: death will be swallowed up in eternity (Isaiah 25:6). That is the goal. In fact, there is even one step beyond, to nullify death retroactively: to bring those who are dead back to life. That is the ultimate Jewish Messianic dream—resurrection; not only to stop death but to reclaim all those who have already died and bring them back to life.

According to classic Judaism this is the ultimate goal of humanity and all humans are called to participate in this process. Obviously, this goal is ambitious and difficult; therefore, one must realize that it will not be accomplished easily or quickly. It may not be accomplished in one lifetime, but the infinite goal can be reached by a series of finite steps. Therefore, all human beings should see themselves as part of the covenantal chain. Each generation advances that covenant as far as possible in one lifetime, with the understanding that it will be taken up by the next generation, and the next, until the final perfection is achieved. The commitment to the covenant is the commitment to pass it on. Each human being must understand that he was not born today. Each is the product of the efforts of the generations that preceded; each one is continuing a human chain that started this journey toward perfection. It has taken enormous stress and effort and sacrifice and building to get this far. Each one plans not to quit until the goal is finally achieved. In short, humans are called to align themselves with the forces of life, with the goal of helping all human beings become the image of God.

Rabbi Joseph B. Soloveitchik has articulated a dimension of the image of God that is important to add to this picture. Soloveitchik says that in the biblical account and Jewish tradition, there are two dimensions of being in the image of God, or like God—two entire modes, one might say, of human existence. One is the mode of being. All people's existence is justified, and has infinite value and uniqueness, simply because they exist. One need not achieve something to justify one's existence. The fact that one is born a human being confers that dignity by right. (This is a fundamental of medical ethics, in the sense that even if a person is sick, or is not a productive member of society, that individual possesses the dignity of being an image of God. No one needs to justify their right to life. The fact that one is not productive at this moment does not take away from one's fundamental value). The quality of being is most developed by relationship. One exists in one's own right; but love, family, relationship to the community, nurture and develop and expand the image of God. In Jewish tradition, relationship to God, as well as to other humans, gives this added dimension of value and of dignity. Indeed, if all the humans in a person's life say that person is nothing, the tradition says there is still the relationship with God as well as God's love; that person has value nonetheless.

The second dimension of human dignified existence is action; it is the mode of control, of achievement, and of mastery of the world that one lives in. Just as God is pure being, justified and powerful and dignified in its own right, so is

God's other dimension, the creative dimension. God is the source of power, creation, life. The human equivalent of being like God is also to show control, achievement, and mastery by dealing with the world, by gaining control over it, by improving it. As one shapes the world, so does one's own sense of dignity and value grow. How does a baby become an effective adult? One of the key elements from the beginning is to reach out to the environment, to play with it, to learn how to manipulate it. In this process of learning control, the baby begins to define himself. Take that same baby and swaddle it, control it, give it no chance of movement or of learning how to cope, and its own development— and value—will be crippled. With the sense of achievement, competence, and coping there accrues a greater dignity for the human being.

Says Soloveitchik: what makes the animal, animal, what makes its existence brute, is that it is helpless; the animal does not have the consciousness or the reason that might enable it to manipulate or control the environment. Therefore, its existence is determined by biology and by the environment which is given to it. It can only adapt; it cannot in any way change reality. What imparts human dignity, then, is power. According to the Bible, *Vatichasrheahu M'at MayElohim* (Psalms 8,6), the human being is "only a little less than God" or "a little less than the angels." The human has the dignity of power—not just the dignity of being like God, but power like God's. Human competence expands human dignity; human power valorizes humans as more and more like God.

An application of the principle: in Jewish tradition, a slave is less than human. By this it is not meant that a slave should be treated as less than human, but rather that being a slave robs one of his human dignity. Therefore, Judaism rejects the notion suggested by Paul in the New Testament that being a slave is irrelevant spiritually. Paul says that whether a slave or a free man, or whether Jew or Gentile, humans are all one in Christ. According to Paul, one's dignity is unaffected by the fact that one is a slave. Jewish tradition asserts that human dignity *is* damaged by the fact that one is a slave. Inability to control one's life, the fact that others control and use and order the person around erodes that person's own dignity and value. In Jewish tradition, the slave was given restitution payments when he was freed to redress the damage done him by his former dependence and loss of dignity.

In the same spirit, Rabbi Joseph B. Soloveitchik (1965) has written that what gives humans dignity, and makes them more and more like God, is the development of technology and science to higher levels. "Man of old could not fight disease, and succumbed in multitudes to yellow fever or any other plague with degrading helplessness could not lay claim to dignity. Only the man who builds hospitals, discovers therapeutic techniques and saves lives is blessed with dignity. Man of the 17th and 18th centuries who needed several days to travel from Boston to New York was less dignified than modern man who attempts to conquer space, boards a plane at New York Airport at midnight and takes several hours later a leisurely walk along the streets of London" (p. 14).

What Rabbi Soloveitchik is saying is that, contrary to the constant emphasis on how medicine or scientific power in general is manipulative and dangerous to human ethics, at its profoundest level, particularly in modern times, it is liberating and religiously inspired. In the process of freeing people from dependency and from slavery to health factors, medical science is the ultimate fulfillment of the Jewish dream, that of the human becoming more and more like God. Thus we are living through the greatest elevation of dignity in human history and doctors are in the forefront of that thrust. Properly understood, every moment spent in medicine is a moment of religious calling and of ethical responsibility, because it is part of that process of perfecting human life. In the same spirit, Maimonides wrote that the specific quality that makes a human 'the image of God' is reason. Reason confers the power that enables man to overcome that biological control and environmental dependency which humans are born into. One must avoid romanticizing mere existence. One must avoid the facile sentimentality of the notion that meditation is somehow more spiritually holy than medication. Physical activity and learning Torah can both be ways of improving the image of God. One must resist the easy supposition that the human being is automatically holier on *Shabbat* than during the week. The weekdays' holiness is, in a way, more challenging, more taxing, more dangerous, but also more liberating and, ultimately, more dignity-conferring. This focus points also to the importance of correcting the human economic, political, and social infrastructure. It is not just medicine that matters, but public health and access to medicine. The economic, political, and social environment—and the bestowal of equality on humans—is part of the religious challenge and of the ultimate dream. Economic productivity, medical technology, as well as human relationship and spiritual exercises, are all part of the religious obligation.

In Genesis, the human was placed in the Garden of Eden, to work it and protect it. The margin of plenty in Paradise is part of human dignity and humans respond by respecting nature. Jewish tradition has always sought to give people guaranteed incomes. When the Israelites settled in Israel, each family was given a piece of land. They were given interest-free loans so they wouldn't lose the land if they had a bad crop. The land was recycled back to individual families in the Jubilee Year. In Messianic times, the Bible says, human beings will have their own land, their own vine, their own fig tree (Micah 4.4); if you will, their own guarantee of dignity.

III

All in all, work, productivity, and medical power constitute a religious calling. But the key to constructive use of power is partnership. Thus one should glorify the use of technology and creativity to free human beings from dependency. The other side of the coin is the notion of protecting the world even as one works [in biblical language, "to work it and protect it" (Genesis 2,15)]. The key is the concept of partnership and not just power for its own sake. The Bible which commands humans to shape the world and conquer it turns around and demands respect for that world. The Torah puts limits on what humans can do to that world. The classic limit is *Shabbat* (the Sabbath). The human who is commanded to work and maximize power all week long is asked to renounce that power on *Shabbat*. *Shabbat* reminds humans that that same power and control which is so crucial to dignity and to spiritual perfection is also the great danger; it may get out of control. The human, who is meant to be more and more like God, becomes confused and begins to think of himself *as* God. The human being who is called upon to acquire maximum power forgets that power itself must be controlled.

One can compare this to the growth process. Growth is the law of life. When an animal stops growing, when the cells stop reproducing, this is the beginning of death. Ultimately, the total cessation of growth is in fact death. Yet if growth gets out of control, if it metastasizes and no longer respects limits or participation in an organic process, growth becomes cancer which also kills.

Shabbat is an attempt to structure an ethical counterbalance to the affirmation of power and human perfection. Similarly, the human body can be perfected through circumcision, but the body as it is now also has dignity and value. One must respect one's own body and its existence. There must be a time set aside for accepting the body—and nature itself—and simply living with it. That is the ethical counterbalance to the manipulation, control, and shaping which is the other human responsibility.

The *Shabbat* itself, when humans are told not to work, is an affirmation of creaturehood which is the counterbalance to the creator role which the Torah affirms all week long. One gives up the creative power for a day. God is the creator; the human is like God by creating and shaping and building the world, 6 days out of every week. On the *Shabbat* day, humans remind themselves that they are not God. They exist as creatures, not as creators.

The definition of the work prohibited on *Shabbat* was taken from two primary models. One was the Holy Temple or *Mishkan,* the Tabernacle itself. The work done in the Tabernacle became the prototype of the kind of work that is prohibited on *Shabbat*. When we analyze those types of work, it is the work involved in planting and harvesting and developing food, and cooking it; in making clothes and weaving them; in short, it is the work of civilization itself. It turns out that the work which is "holy," which one is supposed to give up on *Shabbat,* is in fact modeled after the actual work done to create human civilization.

To put it another way, the tradition is conveying that when people work in civilization, they are doing work in God's Temple. Just as the priest who came into the Temple did God's work by working in the Holy Tabernacle, so a doctor who comes into his office daily is doing God's work, which is perfecting life and guaranteeing its triumph. Thus there is a dialectic in Judaism: power is affirmed, but respect for that which already exists is also affirmed. Holiness consists of shaping and perfecting the world, of developing all the possibilities in life and eliminating sickness, and ultimately hoping to eliminate death, while at the same time respecting and enhancing the life that is.

One must then seek not only to overcome the weakness of life and reshape it, one must also learn to accept life as it is. For the 25 hours of *Shabbat,* one makes no attempt whatsoever to change life. One learns to accept life's rhythms. To apply this concept to the medical rhythm, part of the rhythm is manipulation, control, learning to master life and perfect it. The other aspect is developing the humility to know that a doctor is not God, that a doctor is not infinitely the master; therefore the doctor must learn also to respect what is. The doctor must learn to work with the rhythms of the body and not just to change them, to work with the environment as it is and not just to create superior artificial environments. The practice of medicine, as of humanness, is the art of harnessing the dialectic of being and doing; of accepting what is, at its fullest, but simultaneously trying to change it and perfect it.

The first act one does at the end of *Shabbat* is the *Havdalah* ceremony—the separation ceremony—that has at its heart a display of human technology: lighting a fire. This act is an affirmation, lest anybody think that the *Shabbat* is a denial of human competence, a reflection of God's "jealousy" of human power. Compare the Prometheus myth, in which the human who stole fire from the gods is punished forever; the gods are furious because fire represents human independence from divine control. In Judaism, the first act after the *Shabbat* ends is to light not just one wick, but a multiple wick; one must light not just a light, but a fire powerful enough to heat, to provide radiant energy. Humanly-created fire is the symbol of human liberation, of human technology. It is the symbol of how humans are no longer dependent on their physical environment, but can change it and shape it for their own dignity and value.

The element of dialectical interplay between power and partnership is the covenantal model for medical ethics as well. On the one hand, its implication is to become more and more like God. People ask: what are the limits? The covenantal response is that the limit is nonexistent. I submit that the fear of genetic engineering, the fear of medical control, is in part derived from the inherited ethic of powerlessness, whereby there is deemed something sacrilegious in our ability to gain control over life.

This can be compared to the initial religious attitudes toward birth control. In Jewish tradition, as in Catholic tradition, there is a great deal of resistance to birth control. Part of that resistance is legitimate; it is an attempt to stress the priority of creating life. This is the human calling; the only way to overcome death is by creating life.

On the other hand, the great fear of medicine, experiments, and technology—as of birth control—bespeaks the inherited fear that grew out of an ethic of powerlessness. When humans were powerless to control their own lives, it appeared that God's greatness lay in the control of humans; God's unlimited power in contrast with human powerlessness. There is a kind of residual feeling that the new power is somehow overweening. This fear fails to perceive the covenantal model, which is the model of *partnership*. The world will not be perfected without full human help. Therefore neither birth control nor human technology is sacrilegious.

What are the limits? In principle, the answer is: no limits short of overcoming death. Anything that can advance in this direction is a legitimate outgrowth and a legitimately ethical enterprise. There is one crucial qualification. If the process of liberation gets out of control and persuades the human being to become God, then it is pathological. Power turns into idolatry; this is the ultimate sin in the eyes of

Judaism. Idolatry confuses the human, who is *like* God, *with* God. The human who seeks to be God becomes not God but an idol or demon.

IV

Let us apply all this specifically to medicine. From the beginning the tradition calls medicine a *mitzvah*. This is derived from a verse in Exodus: *ve-rapo yerapay,* "he shall heal" (Exodus 21:19) means that the physician is *commanded* to heal; that it is a *mitzvah*. The very act of healing is a religious enterprise and a religious act. (Now one knows why so few doctors go to *shul* or church. They are too busy being religious. This is said with some irony, of course. It is more likely an example of spiritual metastasis in which the *doing* part often begins to overrun the *being* part. However, there is a certain logic to such a view).

In fulfilling this commandment, physicians are on the side of the Lord. The obvious condition is that the power be used as part of the commitment to be on the side of life itself.

Medicine has to be on the side of life. That may appear a truism. Yet, some forty years ago, SS doctors were in charge of the selections at Auschwitz, in which hundreds of thousands were sent to their death. Doctors were involved in human experimentation at that time. For the most part, that "experimentation" was in fact nothing more than experimentation with death, rather than with life. In Germany in the 1930s, medical doctors experimented on the mentally retarded to develop the very process of gassing which became the preferred method of mass killing of Jews during the Holocaust. This is precisely the challenge of the dialectic. On the one hand, unlimited power is a religious calling. On the other hand, one must have no illusions: such power is available for evil and destruction.

What of nuclear energy itself? On the one hand, it is an incredible achievement of unparalleled power, and it gives access to the ultimate power. One can envision the possibilities to be achieved through nuclear power: freedom from dependence on nature itself. But that same power, cancerously developed, translates into nuclear weapons that can wipe out all of existence. One must solve this paradox not by evading power, but by articulating it as a partnership. One must conceive of power as part of the fact that humans are like God. But humans are not God; therefore, they must have reverence for life. Humans have no right to wipe out life or to endanger it. The way to approach genetic engineering is not to hesitate about the enterprise in the first place, but to exercise the kind of *controls* that make sure one does not lose respect for what *is*. One must not allow the technology to get out of control.

That fundamental limit, the dialectical balance, is the rest of medical ethics. One objective is to bring out the image of God in others by liberating them from sickness and weakness. At the same time, the doctor must recognize, as he deals with humans, that they may each have their own image of God.

The Bible teaches that an all-powerful God who wants humans to become perfect makes a final discovery, that God cannot make them perfect. Why? Because that attempt in itself would be a violation of human dignity and value. If God, using all of God's power, made a person perfect, that person would be a puppet, not a human. A human would be a child's toy which God made by using overwhelming force. The Bible describes how God, starting with the dream of perfection, put two perfect human beings down in a paradise, or a perfect setting. It turned out, however, that in that setting they were entirely dependent and infantile. It is only after they sin that their maturity as full human beings develops. God's initial reaction when humans sinned was the threat to wipe them out (Genesis 2:17). But the Lord relented out of respect for human growth.

In trying to perfect humanity, God does wipe out all of humanity in the Flood. Then God makes a pledge. Unlimited power—even God's—is not possible, if one wishes to reconcile power with the dignity and value of life itself. The conclusion is an act of covenant. God makes a covenant, first with Noah, and only later with the Jewish people. God agrees to control his own power, to limit it, in order to make possible some sort of human participation. In the cosmic process this partnership and growth are necessary if humans are to achieve their full dignity.

To apply this model to medical ethics, the *halakhic* dialectic suggests that to be on the side of life, one must in some way take into account the dignity of life and the dignity of the live subject, namely the patient. The patient, who is the subject of the doctor's overwhelming power, is also an image of God. Therefore, the physician must always be careful that in the exercise of power, during which he has become like God, he respects the dignity of the patient in his very existence as an image of God. The patient must not be treated simply as a subject of aggrandizement, or as an object of manipulation. The very act of human healing, which is in a sense acting like God, involves the recognition of the image of God in others. This is the doctor's covenantal commitment.

Jewish tradition says that in medical ethics, as in all ethics, life comes first. Saving a life is the ultimate calling. Perfecting life is the second stage. Saving life overrides all commandments in the tradition, except three. These three illuminate the doctor's role.

One is murder. To murder somebody else is wrong because one is degrading life. There is no right to kill an innocent person, even to save one's own life, because the very act of killing that other person, if innocent, degrades all of life.

Secondly, the tradition says that stopping certain forms of sexual immorality, such as incest, overrides the commandment to save life. The rabbis felt that, given the fundamental importance of the sexual function and the parental function, to permit such immorality would disturb the basic human pattern. Compare the child-abuse pattern; children who are abused are likely, in turn, to become abusers. If the fundamental structure of sexuality in a parent-child relationship is disturbed, basic human dignity is endangered. Therefore, one has to fight that possibility at all costs, even unto death.

The third case is idolatry. The rabbis ruled that one should die rather than commit idolatry. The rabbis touch here upon a great truth. If human beings exaggerate and aggrandize themselves to the degree that they set themselves up as God, then they are truly idolaters, because all other humans will thereby become so degraded as to become less than human. Therefore, it is worth dying if one is on the side of life; one must die rather than let idolatry triumph. There is that thin line of the dialectic. On the one hand, humans are commanded to become more and more like God. If they cross that line and become God, they will not enhance the quality of life; they will degrade it.

One may see this in the evidence of the Holocaust. For the first time in human history, one saw total human power, total control over others. It was power in its idolatrous form. In the Holocaust, Hitler was God, or Mengele was God or Eichmann was God; they had total control over life and death. In this form, power turned out to be demonic and cancerous rather than life-giving. Dr. Joseph Mengele, the doctor who was in charge of inmate selections at Auschwitz,

scheduled a special selection every Yom Kippur, on the Day
of Atonement. On the day that Jews pray and say that God
decides who shall live and who shall die, Mengele held a
special selection and said in public, "*I* decide who shall live
and who shall die."

The danger of unleashed power that becomes truly idolatrous is that it becomes an ultimate source of death, and
not of life. That is the potential and the danger in medicine—
as it is in all of human power. The tradition says that if the
doctor wants to be a source of life rather than death, the
key to doing good rather than evil is the concept of covenant
or partnership. The physician who respects the body will
bear in mind that a medication which saves a patient can
also, by the very fact of interference, cause side-effects
which are disruptive and destructive. Therefore, the good
healer is one who works maximally with the minimal intervention. Just as limited biological pesticides would be preferable to strong chemicals that destroy the environment, so
is the intervention within the patient maximized by working
with the patient's body rather than overpowering it—even
for good.

Secondly, the patient himself must have a role in therapy.
The patient is in the image of God; then the greater the role
in the patient's own therapy, the greater the patient's own
dignity. The greater the patient's say in those matters which
affect the patient's life, the more Godlike is the patient. Such
medical approaches as informed consent and sharing information on decision making, wherever possible, are part of
the recognition that the patient's sense of his own capabilities is part of the cure. If doctor makes the patient totally
dependent and totally infantilized, the patient is less likely
to respond well and less likely to be healed.

Patients who have a will to live do better than patients
who have lost their will to live. This concept is true across
the boards—before it gets to that extreme form of will to

live. In the case of Barney Clark, the artificial heart recipient, Clark was chosen to become the first such recipient in part because he showed considerable psychological strength and balance. Nevertheless some weeks after his operation, he only infrequently made eye contact with others in the hospital. One member of Clark's medical team said he believed this was Dr. Clark's response to the humiliation of lying in bed undressed much of the time, completely dependent, unable to speak without an effort. When Dr. Clark's condition was improving, his doctors and nurses noted that he made more eye contact with them. He started conversations with the staff more often and addressed them more directly.

It also developed that Clark showed a persistent state of confusion for many days following a number of seizures. After being repeatedly asked about Clark's confusion, the university vice president said to the reporter in question, "Stand up here, let us take off your clothes, make you unable to speak very well, put needles and tubes in you, have night indistinguishable from day over a several-week period, and then I'll ask if by any chance you are frustrated or confused."

The reality is that the sixty-two-year-old retired dentist's experience was not so different, in many respects, from that of others in intensive care units for long periods. What about the basic structure of medicine, or offices, or hospitals themselves? What about the extent to which, in a medical center situation, not only are the doctors indifferent technicians rather than compassionate professionals, but all too many times staff members are less than sensitive to patients needs? Nurses, clerks, secretaries, and orderlies all affect the patient's self-esteem. When a patient is lying in a hospital and there are dirty clothes on the floor instead of in a bin— even trivial details like this when patients are being examined can have demoralizing effects. When a patient is asked questions, how the question is asked and the conditions under which the doctor is going through the questioning, can have an enormous effect on the patient. This kind of sensitivity is part of the concept of a role for the patient in therapy, and part of the respect for that patient.

One must fully recognize the fact that one cannot be purely idealistic in medicine. A covenantal ethic of medicine, perforce, is an ethics of power. But it is crucial to that whole ethic that the doctors see this element, and respect it, too. The loss of will, and anxiety and weakness in the patient lead to less effective response. Doctors must recognize the human being as a psychic being, not just a chemical being. Doctors do not always have to resort to chemicals; they must be willing to play a psychic role, too. Doctors are becoming more and more aware that the distinctions between psychosomatic medicine and regular medicine are eroding; one translates into the other. Psychic responses translate into hormones, or into chemical receptors in the brain, just as chemical receptors translate into emotions.

All of this ethical instruction is ultimately an ethic of power, not of powerlessness. Here is where I think ethics can learn from medicine, as much as medicine can learn from the ethics. In an ethic of power, the first principle is that power must be used. It is a *mitzvah,* a religious ethical response and fulfillment, to use maximum power to achieve maximum perfection of life.

Secondly, an ethic of power (rather than powerlessness), operates in the real world. Medical triage, obviously, is such a situation. In many cases, the real choice is not perfection, but the choice of the lesser evil of the two. These judgments are inescapable—and proper. In the real world, in the use of power, "good" inevitably has side effects which are bad. The real tension comes in balancing these side effects; if the good outweighs the bad, one is entitled to act. Where real good can be accomplished, acting is the more ethical response; failure to act is unethical.

If, in order to protect one's self, one does not use a certain medication even when its good outweighs the bad, if a physician calculates that the side effects may be harmful, and using the right medicine will make him vulnerable to criticism (or for that matter, being struck back at through a malpractice suit) then the physician is being unethical by not acting. The only people who can be perfect are those who have never used power and never helped anyone. The only thing that is more immoral than excessive intervention is no intervention whatsoever.

Show me a good doctor and I will show you somebody who has buried patients. If they had not done that, they would not have saved all the lives that they did. And this has to be part of the honesty and the integrity of society's ethical judgments as well as the judgments of how to handle a situation. To use less power than necessary, or to *resist* the development of power out of excessive fear is a form of ethical abuse and of not taking humanity seriously. If there is a capacity for good, it should be developed.

The original birth control prohibition in Jewish law reflects the fear that human control over who shall be created, who shall be given life, is somehow robbing God of his power. What is *really* involved in birth control is an ethical trade-off: the quality of life versus the quantity of life. It is necessary to know that quantity is important. It's also essential to know that quality matters. If the marriage needs more time, if the mother needs more time or cannot handle the number of children, then it is ethical *not* to have the child rather than to have it. That is the balancing act that has to be undertaken.

The same holds true on questions of abortion. There is a profound ethical truth behind all those who oppose abortion.

It is important for doctors to see it; when ending life, even during this prenatal stage, becomes casual, there will be a weakening of respect for all of life. Yet abortion can also be an act of taking responsibility for the quality of life of a mother; it can be the difference between life and a blasted life.

In Jewish tradition, the ideal life-style is vegetarianism—in the long run. When one kills animals, one weakens respect for human life itself. Yet, the tradition permits meat to be eaten by Jews, precisely because it realized that if one protects the animal's life, above all else, one is going to end up in a situation where sacred cows walk the streets undisturbed and well-fed, while humans starve to death every day. That paradoxical outcome of Hindu vegetarianism is the same risk tied to the absolute position on abortion. One must continually understand the dialectic of partnership and the dialectic of ethical responsibility; one must juggle and not set up an either/or as a simple automatic responsibility.

The conflict over autopsy in recent times follows the same pattern. The traditional objection to autopsy was respect for human life. No doctor should underestimate the fact that if humans are to be respected as valuable in their own right—not because they are useful, but in their own right—then one of the most powerful ways to do so is to show respect for humans even when they are dead. If one uses a dead person, that is a way of saying that human beings are only valuable when they are useful. Even when a person is dead, one wants to use the person in some way.

This may sound extreme, but recall the Holocaust experience. The Nazis, after they killed the Jews, turned their ashes into fertilizer and soap. They spread the roads with the ashes of Jews in wintertime because they wanted to show that the Jews were things, and not people. They had the right to use them and use them up, to the last particle.

However, the other side of the coin is that the *purpose*

for respecting the dead is a respect for *life*—to show that life is precious. Therefore, one has a right to use the dead when it increases life and the quality of life. Hence the ethical necessity of autopsies. If an autopsy can lead to a medical breakthrough or to new understanding, then it is a *requirement*. A family that hesitates, or a rabbi who says no, is not being ethical or religious. This is being sacrilegious—placing a dead body ahead of a living person.

How does one resolve these tensions? That is exactly what covenantal morality is about. It is the partnership of mastery of being with respect for being; the struggle to strike a balance is what counts. This covenantal model, then, is the ultimate model behind medicine in this time. This is the challenge to doctors: to develop their own capacity medically, to realize every moment of research is in fact sacred. When one approaches research, one must approach it with all the reverence that one brings to a special occasion.

"Holiness" means "uniquely special." Every act of research, every act of treatment is unique and holy, precisely because it is part of that struggle for respect for life and perfection of life. Precisely because it is holy, one must approach it with consciousness, with reverence for being, and with a sense of humility in one's own limits. This balance of power should be welcomed by all concerned. Informed consent is a way of transferring power to the patient. Professional peer review is a covenantal act. Malpractice suits are a form of ethical behavior in this sense: when doctors fail to exercise their own control, then malpractice suits are a form of ethical corrective of the balance of power. It is precisely that pressure that forces some recognition or sensitivity, some awareness of limits.

The complication besetting all these issues is that in creating a new balance of power, one often creates new evils. All power has inescapable side effects. Malpractice suits spawn lawyers out to make a fortune, and therefore looking for trouble; one sees the exploitation of minor errors for major settlements. These are all abuses. But, in a very real sense, the struggle to create countervailing force and prevent excessive abuses is part of the covenantal process, too.

This challenge of medical ethics in our times is truly of an unprecedented magnitude. On the one hand, doctors are in the forefront of humanity, fostering dignity and the triumph of life itself. One can truly see, in the breakthroughs in bio-engineering and medicine occurring today, the beginning of the recognition that life may yet triumph. On the other hand, the key to all this becoming a triumph of life, and not of death, is the ability of doctors to develop a covenantal model of self-limitation. Doctors must work with society to create a balance of power; and they must work with themselves to create a climate of respect for human beings as well.

All this may sound exaggerated or extreme. The Jewish claim that life will totally triumph over death sounds absurd on the face of it. Who should be more conscious of the absurdity than doctors who live with death every day? Yet note the following paradox: Every human being who ever lived, except those who are still alive at this moment, has died. This would appear to prove that death cannot lose. In fact, that is false. Thanks to the power of love and of human commitment to create life and perfect it, there is more life in the world, more perfect forms of life, and more access to health today, than ever before in human history.

Before they died, humans saw themselves as part of a process of life. They created life; they had their own children; they perfected life in the form of developing science and medicine and other forms of technological respect for life. Thus, before they died humans so increased life that humanity today is living in a period of overwhelming expansion of life. One can see on the horizon the possibility of its triumph. Doctors who stand in a moment of history parallel to creation might learn a lesson and walk in the footsteps of a God who at such a moment undertook a covenantal commitment to limit God's power. At the moment of breakthrough, the recognition of the unlimited potential for redeeming life should be the final incentive for doctors to accept the challenge of turning from power to love. This is the impetus for doctors to voluntarily surrender one-sided total power and truly take up the challenge of a convenantal ethic.

10

Jewish Medical Ethics and Law

Rabbi Emanuel Rackman, Ph.D.

*I*n Jewish medical ethics there are very few black and white answers; there are mostly gray ones. Therefore, in the final analysis, a rabbi can very rarely decide for the family, or the doctor, or the hospital administrator. Ideally, there should be consultation among, and input from, all the participants: the patient (if possible), family, doctors, and rabbis. If all parties accept this premise, we will see that even the person who does not know Jewish law and is no expert at all in *halakhah*, can contribute significantly to the ethical decision that is to be implemented; and the final decision, even if the rabbi does not concur in it, may turn out to be one which superficially conforms with one or another *halakhic* precedent or *halakhic* authority on which a rabbi might have relied.

Mine is a minority opinion among rabbis, certainly among Orthodox rabbis. I have been referred to as the leading maverick in the Orthodox rabbinate. Actually, I believe that I am very, very traditional. However, I have studied not only the *halakhah*—the laws, the rules—but also the *ha-*

lakhic process. I try to describe that process as it is, and decision making is a process in which many factors must play a role. I try to tell the truth about the *halakhic* process, and while I see some value in mythologizing some of its aspects, I also want to contribute to its demythologization.

In every system—the political system, the economic system—there is a certain value in creating myths. It is often easier to communicate ideas through myths. I am not talking about Greek myths. I am talking about slogans which convey or encapsulate a system's basic ideas, but which upon closer examination do not really conform with the facts. So, while I feel that I am very traditional, I nonetheless think we will appreciate the *halakhah* more if we understand its process. We must understand that we can all play a part in this process; not as ignoramuses, but as people who, with heart and soul and intelligence, apply themselves to it.

There is a story told about a man who, after being importuned by his wife for many, many months, finally decided to clean out the attic. He did it, and then confided to a friend: "You know, I did a stupid thing. In the attic there was a family Bible. My wife wanted me to throw out everything, so I threw that out, too. Now I realize that on the frontispiece of that Bible there were the big letters, G-U-T-E-N." The friend exploded, "You idiot! You probably burned a Gutenberg Bible. The last copy of a Gutenberg Bible sold for about $40,000 at auction, and you went ahead and took that Gutenberg Bible and burned it!" The man replied, "Well, I don't think my copy would have brought a cent, because it had glosses written all over the margins by some character named Martin Luther!"

I am one who is very much committed to the Bible—and to the Oral Law—which are the glosses have been written throughout the centuries. Because I am so committed to this, I see a process taking place, and this process is dynamic. It fascinates me, and it is the picture of this process that I want to convey, and perhaps show how it can be applied to medical ethics, which also evolved. There are no black and white answers, but gray answers; heart-rending deliberation, soul-searching deliberation—but with the participation of all involved, especially in the implementation of the decision.

By demythologizing, what do we mean? Some Orthodox rabbis say that Jewish law never changes; that it is fixed, immutable. They know this isn't true, but perhaps they say it because they feel that this is in itself creates a value: that people should not get used to the idea that Jewish law can be changed. Changes are often requested by people whose motivation is simply selfish. They want a way to justify what they want to do, with no consideration of the impact of that decision on themselves, on society, and those close to them.

Therefore, Rabbi Joseph B. Soloveitchik, the great mentor of orthodox rabbis in our generation, suggests that instead of saying *halakhah* does not change, we should perhaps speak in terms of innovation in *halakhah,* or of creativity in an immutable *halakhah*. This is what I mean when I suggest demythologizing. It is only a matter of semantics. We must recognize that there is a dynamic process going on all the time. It is conceivable that one day Jews may do according to the *halakhah* what they once could not do; and that they may not be able to do, according to the *halakhah,* what they once could.

The first example of this is smoking. A century or two ago, before smoking became the habit of so many, one questioned whether one could smoke on *Yom Tov*. Smoking on the Sabbath, of course, was forbidden, but the *halakhic* sources differed with regard to smoking on *Yom Tov*. One is allowed to use fire on holidays (that don't occur on the Sabbath) if cooking is involved, which everybody needs for survival. Cigarette smoking wasn't considered in that category until smoking became so prevalent that it was permitted even on *Yom Tov*. Today, it might very well be that that has changed; and there already is a complete prohibition with regard to smoking.

Many things were once prohibited to an extent that is virtually indescribable, such as the taking of usury, or even of any kind of interest. Do I have to tell you to what extent Jews over the last thousand years have broken with that, and have sought all kinds of subterfuges to get around it? True, there was economic necessity during the Middle Ages, but think of interest rates today in Israel, and even at Orthodox banks. Banks owned by Jews are taking 80 percent and 90 percent interest per annum. Thus we see that there were things once prohibited that today are permitted, and people don't bat an eyelash.

How does such change take place? There are many ways. One way in which the legal process develops, or allows for creativity and innovation, is through logic. Logic is a very important factor in law. As a matter of fact, there are three factors that play a part in all legal development: One is logic; the second is the sense of justice; and the third concerns the needs of society. All three elements play a part in Jewish law that there's no escaping. This is true of all legal systems and of the *halakhic* system as well.

A logical approach would be, for example, to ask "Can we use fire on the Sabbath?" Certainly not: It is prohibited in the Bible. Is electricity fire? One can use the logical method; you can try to define fire. The Talmud did. Fire involves burning coals. Therefore, what is prohibited by the Bible is burning *coal,* not hot metal. In this century, Rabbi Goren said, "Electricity is not prohibited biblically, because it is not fire." The flow of electric current through tungsten is not fire; this is hot metal and no more, therefore its use is not biblically prohibited.

This is the method of logic. There's no consideration, in this method, of larger questions: What is the purpose of the

Sabbath? What are its goals? There is no consideration of social needs, or the ease, or lack of it, with which one can produce fire. You start with a definition, you proceed with that definition, and QED, as the geometer does, as the mathematician does, to a conclusion.

The second approach by which law develops, a sense of justice, plays an important part. Most people are unaware of it. Lawyers speak of it as natural law. Jewish law has great concern with what is known as natural law, which simply means one's sense of justice.

For example, we are familiar with the biblical story how God was about to destroy two cities, and Abraham argued with Him: God, how can you do this? You, Who are supposed to be the Judge of all the earth? How can you be so unjust as to destroy the righteous with the wicked?—And thus starts the first dialogue: Abraham bargaining with God. If there are fifty righteous people, will you do it? If there are forty, thirty, twenty, ten? And they couldn't find ten to save the city.

What was the basis of Abraham's argument? He was not arguing on the basis of the fact that the Ten Commandments had already been given. After all, there was no Torah yet; he was the first Jew. Rather, he was arguing from a sense of justice: Will the Judge of all the earth not do justice? This is what we mean by natural law.

There is a much more sophisticated illustration which shows the humanitarian character of Jewish law. Thousands of years before Abraham Lincoln spoke of the Union not being able to exist half slave and half free, there was such a phenomenon in Jewish law as a person who was half slave and half free.

Say a man owns a slave. The man dies, and two sons survive him. One son emancipates the slave, so the slave is half free; the other son refuses to emancipate. Thus there is a man who is half slave and half free. What does one do in that case?

There arose the school of Hillel—the famous Hillel for whom even the non-Jewish world had such profound respect, because it identifies with what is regarded as the humanitarian aspects of Hillel's thought—which said, "What's the difficulty? Let him work for the master to whom he is still bonded. Let him work for that master Sunday, Tuesday, and Thursday; and on Monday, Wednesday, and Friday, he'll work for himself. On the Sabbath, he's not allowed to work at all."

Then spoke the school of Shamai, the so-called strict school, that was supposed to be the school without a heart. "How can you do that to the man," asked Shamai. "It's true that you've solved the needs of the master; the master who still owns half of him can enjoy his services. But what about the slave? He can't marry a free woman because he's half slave. He can't marry a slave woman because he's half free. What is he to do with his life, with his humanity, with his right to have a family, and establish himself in society?"

Shamai came up with a beautifully simple solution; one that isn't based on scriptual text, nor even on logic. For on the basis of text, there is no requirement in the Torah that a man be married; he can be fruitful and multiply without marriage. Why, then, insist on this slave's "right" to marry?

But the school of Shamai declared that the thing to do would be to force the master who still has him enslaved to emancipate him. The slave will then work for himself all week as a wholly freed man, and from his earnings repay the master who was reluctant to free him. Thus, the half owner doesn't lose his property rights, but the slave can still be a human being, exercising all of his human rights.

This is the sense of justice that permeates Jewish law. *Bet Hillel,* the school of Hillel, admitted that the school of Shamai was right. They confessed their error and the decision was unanimous.

Jewish law was always responsive to social needs: to those of Jewish society and those of society in general. Although there is much written in modern Jewish literature on this topic, I shall briefly cite just two examples.

The first is the prohibition, in biblical law, against taking interest. But subsequently there developed a need for Jewish law to permit Jews to become moneylenders—one of the few occupations allowed them in the Middle Ages. Ways were found to subvert—to employ that term—the biblical law. Similarly, there is a biblical rule with regard to the abolition of debts in the seventh year. The result was that during the other 6 years Jews would not lend money to each other, for the debt might be cancelled. There had to be a resort to a legal fiction to encourage Jews to lend money to each other, or panic would have ensued.

Another example is a relatively modern procedure which is not much respected by Jews, but, when properly understood, ought to evoke respect. On the Passover holiday Jews may not own *hametz* (leavened bread or cakes). Therefore, they resort to a legal fiction; they sell it to a non-Jew. This tradition didn't come about because Jews in those days had freezers, and were stocking them up long in advance with bagels; it came about because Jews were the innkeepers for most of the Eastern European lords of the manor. Jews had the liquor licenses, and had to account to the *paritz* (the lord) with regard to the sale of liquor.

What would happen the day before Passover? The Jews couldn't take the liquor and destroy it. Although there may have been enough of their contemporaries available to drink it, the Jews would still have to pay the nobleman for it. Therefore if Jews were to continue in this occupation, the rabbis had to create a device whereby Jews, without violating Jewish law, could continue to pursue their livelihood.

Thus there was always a positive response in Jewish law to social needs, together with a sense of justice, and certainly with logic playing its role as well. The principles and the underlying values do not change; the rules change. Call it innovation, call it creativity; the law is dynamic. To think of it as unchangeable, immutable is a myth.

The second myth is that the *halakhic* expert is totally objective. It is true that the *halakhic* expert may not say, "I am deciding the case this way, because I want this to be the outcome." One must be judicious in making any kind of a legal decision; in no court do judges say they're deciding a case in a certain manner because they want it that way. The decision of the judges, at least superficially, from the point of view of the myth of the judicial process, must be objective; they must do what they do in the name of justice.

But can anyone be that totally objective? The famous Supreme Court Justice Cardozo wrote in his book, *The Nature of the Judicial Process,* that it is inevitable that a judge will have his own personal philosophy. For example, does a prominent, successful attorney for the railroads really think that the owners and operators of this country's railroads were or are thieves? He undoubtedly has an affection for them; he's going to take their word more readily than he will take the word of someone who is not connected with the industry of which he is a part.

A real-life example of this phenomenon occurred at Yeshiva University which I once attended. In the early 1950s, the school undertook to draft its students for the military chaplaincy in the United States. A group of students protested; they objected on the theory that drafting students to become chaplains in the military establishment might one day involve them in the desecration of the Sabbath or in funeral procedures which some of them might deem *halakhically* prohibited.

It was decided to let Rabbi Soloveitchik resolve the case. He was asked whether it was permitted for the university, in effect, to say to the students: "We will not ordain you unless you spend 2 years in the chaplaincy serving the United States of America." Rabbi Soloveitchik wrote a brilliant, 20-page, single-spaced responsum, permitting it. In the beginning of the responsum he admitted that he felt the need to resolve this problem affirmatively. He searched and searched, and found a basis on which it could be done.

This was not being objective—to start off with one's conclusion, and then say, "I found the way to accomplish what I want"; but he was honest. The *halakhic* expert who is honest will say, "I tried my best to be as objective as possible, but no one is so saintly; if we were angels, perhaps we could do it."

In chapter 2 of the *Guide to the Perplexed,* Maimonides discusses what it was that Adam and Eve destroyed in the Garden of Eden. Until they ate the fruit, says Maimonides, all their ethical judgments were based upon pure reason. What happened by their eating the fruit was that a third factor came in—emotion, will; and these corrupted man. If man could always be rational, perhaps there would be none of the problems that we have today.

It is important for the *halakhic* expert occasionally to say, as Rabbi Soloveitchik did, "I wanted the result I found." He does not impeach his credibility by being honest. He said that he tried to be objective, but acknowledges the natural fact that no human being can be 100 percent objective.

On many occasions I have had the opportunity to argue with rabbis who were opposed to some of the claims of the feminist movement. I said to them, in essence: What's your attitude toward women? If you're as fond of them as I am, you'll make one response. But if you really have no respect for them, if you think their place is in the home, in the kitchen, raising children, then you will have another response to many of the issues that come from the feminist movement. It's a person's attitude that frequently determines the conclusion.

A third myth is that *halakhah* is not influenced by current conditions and circumstances; of course, it *is.* It does not change solely *because* of current needs and circumstances, but it is responsive *to* them. Sometimes it will make radical changes through a response, which is geared to needs and circumstances having an ethical dimension.

One of the most classic instances is the case, in a somewhat obscure *mishnah,* involving the price of fowl. The cost of fowl and other birds rose so high that women who were obligated to bring offerings to the temple (in order to be admitted to the temple on festivals) couldn't afford the required offerings. Some of them were required to bring four or five such offerings, and the dealers in fowl raised the prices so high that the women couldn't afford to buy them. What did the rabbis do? They said they would dispense with the need for bringing many offerings; one would suffice. The prices immediately collapsed. That was response to an economic crisis.

Judges, even in other judicial systems, will rarely spell out the need and the circumstances that warranted a particular response. There is what is called a crypto-legal method. Logic is used. The decision is justified on the basis of precedents. One distinguishes between this and that precedent, but essentially it's a sociological, or psychological, or, as I would claim, a teleological need that prompts you to do what you do.

The fourth myth is that the *halakhah* is immutable, and never transcends its own rules. The fact is, there are instances in history when the law was completely transcended—when the rabbis declared, "This is a need which prompts us to say that the *halakhah* is in abeyance." Referred to here are biblical rules—not simply rabbinical rules—being disregarded.

My good friend Rabbi Walter Wurzburger, editor of the well-known Orthodox periodical *Tradition,* gives these situations a beautiful name. He calls them covenantal imperatives. These are situations which compel Jews to say, because of the inescapable dynamic of their very covenant, "We cannot obey the law." It is as if a man under contract to someone else might say, "I know that I am bound by this contract, but by the demands of the contract itself, I see my moral and ethical right to abrogate the contract." This concept was implemented in at least one case involving the use of the word *Shalom*. *Shalom,* the name of God, is used very freely, simply in greeting. It is a common phrase on the lips of Jews. Yet a commandment in the Torah states, "Thou shalt not bear the name of God in vain." Despite this, the rabbis permitted Jews to greet each other with the word *Shalom,* which apparently had become a customary greeting, something that people of themselves had created. The rabbis didn't try to stop this trend. They simply said, in effect: God certainly would have wanted this. Even though He prohibited the use of His name in vain, to greet one another in His name serves a covenantal end. When you are doing something for God, you are allowed to violate even the fundamentals of Torah.

There are other illustrations connected with this concept. The famous Rabbi Nissenbaum, who perished in the Holocaust, delivered a sermon on Yom Kippur to the Jews in the death camps. He said there's a difference between Jewish law in the Middle Ages and Jewish law today. In the Middle Ages, the rabbis may have told their congregations that it was their moral duty to be martyrs. For in the Middle Ages, the Christian world (or Moslem world, in some instances) said to the Jew, We want your soul; we want you to become baptized or we want you to accept Mohammed as the Prophet: religious coercion. The only way the Jew could stop himself from being converted was by letting himself by martyred.

Therefore, said Rabbi Nissenbaum, in the Middle Ages it was the Jew's duty to martyr himself for the glory of God. But in the modern age, in the age of Hitler, Hitler didn't want the Jewish soul. Baptism didn't help the Jew save his life. What the Nazi wanted was the Jewish body. He wanted to destroy all the Jewish bodies he could find. Therefore, it became the Jew's duty to save his body, no matter how he did it: escape; pretend to be a priest or a nun.

Men who are today Hasidic rabbis, wearing long caftans, beards, and *payot,* saved their lives by dressing and behaving as Catholic priests. Rabbis were encouraged to do anything to save the human body. Thus there are covenantal imperatives which supersede what might be called the technical rules. It is a crucial moment in the history of the relationship between God and His people that makes one ignore what is written and subscribe to an imperative that transcends the covenant.

These myths—for lack of a better word—should not be discarded. They are important. It is good that people talk about the fixity and immutability of the *halakhah.* Otherwise, many of us might become too radical. We might say that a man can do what he wants; after all, the Rabbis did what they wanted. Therefore it is important to have rules that will at least *deter.* The myths are deterrents for any radical innovation which is only self-serving. But in dealing with a critical situation, one as basic as the life and death of an individual (sometimes even of a society), then one has to call a spade a spade.

Having exposed these "myths," let me offer a positive picture of the *halakhic* process. There are biblical rules and there are rabbinical rules; and there are, in addition to the rules, the principles and the values; and these are quite different. The rules may change. The principles and the values are fairly static, they don't change radically. The *application* of a principle in order to achieve the value, which is fairly firm, and the manner in which this is done, is an interesting area.

Rabbi Soloveitchik discusses this; and I have also written

extensively about it in an essay entitled *The Dialectic and the Halakhah*. There are opposing poles, ideas which are really antinomies. In making the *halakhic* decision, the poles represent absolute values; but one veers between these poles. Sometimes this is like walking a tightrope. It must be done with all the heart, all the soul-searching one can possibly muster, and it frequently involves a rending of the heart.

This is different from Hegel's concept of the thesis. History moves, said Hegel, from acceptance of a thesis to its antithesis; and then, somehow, we achieve a synthesis. The synthesis then becomes a new thesis, which in turn evolves into another antithesis. In Jewish law, by contrast, the principles are firm. When we say, for example, that the body of a man does not belong to the individual but belongs to God, that is a fixed principle. But the rules that we derive *from* it may change from time to time, because there is another "pole."

The other pole pertains to the sanctity of life, the quality of life. There are the needs of general society, and the needs of Jewish society, which may be different. These are poles. The *halakhist* must bear them in mind. We may move from one to the other in making decisions; depending on circumstances, we may favor one pole or the other. Sometimes the decision will be between the poles, and we call that veering between antinomies.

In the case of actual legislation, there are many things that can be done. For example, in the economic sphere, Jewish law is flexible, as one can imagine, and that's because there has been a fundamental principle in Jewish law that a Jewish court or a Jewish legislature can declare property ownerless. In other words, there could be any kind of experimentation in the area of property, and it would be perfectly acceptable.

There is no such thing as the sacred right of property in Jewish law. The majority of the court and the majority of society, if it so desires, can make decisions, distribute ownership. Judaism, in the economic sphere, is generally quite conservative. It does not approve of mass accumulation of wealth, but it also does not favor the communist ideal of complete sharing.

In Jewish family law, there is tremendous flexibility, because it is assumed that all marriages are performed upon the condition that the rabbinical courts approve. There was never any problem in Jewish law, up to about a thousand years ago, in annulling marriages. While it is not heard of today, there *was* such a thing in Jewish law as annulment of marriage. There has been great of liberalism in regard to the law of bastardy, the legitimacy of children. The Israeli press is fond of smearing the image of Jewish law by discussing this issue, always negatively; but actually, the humanitarianism of Jewish law is so evident as always to emerge. It is the most eloquent evidence of the dynamism of Jewish law and its attitude toward the illegitimate.

Only within the last hundred years or less has American law taken a humane point of view with regard to the child who is presumably illegitimate. There was a time when an illegitimate child couldn't even inherit from his or her natural parent. Jewish law is very liberal in this area. The cardinal rule has been that a child is legitimate as long as it has not been born as the result of an adulterous or incestuous relationship. Children born out of wedlock have always been considered legitimate.

The next question the rabbis asked was, how are you going to prove illegitimacy, since most acts of intercourse by a married woman are imputed to her husband? Even if a husband came home after 5 years from the war in Korea (and everybody knew that he was in Korea for those 5 years) and found his wife with a baby three years old, it was considered his baby. His wife could have conceived by artificial insemination.

That is how far the rabbis went. Fifteen hundred to 2,000 years ago, they thought of the possibility of artificial insemination and limited the charge of illegitimacy, based on the fact that the child might have been born through such means, rather than through an adulterous or incestuous relationship. Then there was a final rule that the child must be an absolute, unqualifiedly illegitimate child. If there was any doubt, the rule did not apply. The rabbis thereby practically abolished the stigma of illegitimacy. This offers some illustration of the manner in which Jewish law responded to humanitarian demands, while never changing the law.

The law, however, remained. It was good to propagate a certain fear, or induce a fear, in order to safeguard young girls. Let them have a fear of this, the rabbis were saying; they'll take better care of themselves; they'll be more chaste; they'll be spared much embarrassment. And so, sometimes, even though the ultimate result may be that there will be no sanction, *caution* is induced.

In criminal law, many passages of the Bible were nullified: for example, the law of the wayward child. Again, the rabbis said, this law was propagated only to make children behave. It was also given to teach parents that they can't expect to produce good children if they do not agree on basic ways of running a household. If such a case did occur, the Bible said the child could be punished; but the rabbis said that you couldn't punish the child. If he's under thirteen, he's not responsible for his acts. If he's over thirteen, he doesn't have to obey his parents; he can do what he wants. So, actually, what's the period of time during which you can punish him for being a wayward child?

Capital punishment is a major issue today. Jews had practically abolished it. All of this was part of the dynamic process; but the rules remain. There are certain Rabbinic rules that don't change: the two days of *Rosh Hashanah,* for example, which even most Reform congregations today observe.

There are many factors that went into *halakhic* change and creativity. When we know these factors, then perhaps we can see how they can be applied to medical ethics. The logical method, which has been referred to, is practically of no help here at all. The problems are too new. There are situations which the rabbis never visualized. The *principles* might remain the same; but the *rules* don't apply.

What is the difference between a 40-day pregnancy, a 60-day pregnancy, and a 6-month pregnancy? Nowhere in the Bible is this discussed. Perhaps there are some references to it in the Talmudic literature. Yet today such differentiations can be extremely important.

Rabbi Bleich feels very strongly that where there's a possibility of Tay-Sachs disease in an unborn child, after the relevant tests have been administered, an abortion should not be permitted after a certain period—certainly not after 6 months.

A great authority in Israel—probably the greatest authority on Jewish medical ethics in the world—is Rabbi Waldenberg. He permits such an abortion (in cases involving Tay-Sachs) at any time, even after the sixth month, as long as it does not endanger the life of the mother. This shows how responsive this rabbi is to the quality of life—not simply the *sanctity* of life, but the *quality* of the life to be born.

Rabbi Bleich then mounted a brilliant attack on the decision of Rabbi Waldenberg, pointing out that Rabbi Waldenberg was relying upon a source a century and a half or two centuries old; moreover, that source was a forgery! Nonetheless, Rabbi Waldenberg, conceding that it was a forgery, did not change his opinion. Here lies the interesting point. Though he originally cited the source, he was in fact relying upon his own ethical and moral sense. How he put it was that Jews have accepted that passage as authoritative, although it may have been a mistake. There are things we say in our prayers that were printers' errors, yet we keep on saying them. He didn't choose to change his opinion, and the decision remains. That is not a logical approach, but it is a humane one.

There are many rabbis who favor what might be called the no-risk approach; they don't want to take any chances. They are dealing with God's law, as they see it, and would rather run no risk in making a decision which might offend God, or offend the tradition; they want to play it safe. That is hardly the answer in medical ethics. Nor is history very helpful. What *can* make a difference, however, is, a three-faceted aproach which is sociological, psychological, and teleological. The resort to sociology is important, meaning by sociology concern for the sanctity of life, but at the same time concern for the sanctity, or the needs, of society. The sanctity of life is so important in Jewish law that one cannot visualize Jews ever permitting infanticide. (Such practices are a fact in modern China.) One cannot see its being permitted on the basis of tradition, even if one personally were convinced that it were allowed.

Interestingly, I here quote Bertrand Russell; than whom there hardly could be more of a secularist. Russell was against the religious tradition, and always derided it. In his book, *"Power,"* he wrote, "I've been told by scientists that the day may come when we have to gas millions of babies after they are born. Somehow, I cannot let myself believe that that would have to happen, and I can't see myself agreeing that it will happen." He didn't live to see infanticide become prevalent in China (*Nation,* 237:12-14, July 2, 1983, and *Newsweek,* 103:47, April 30, 1984).

I see no possibility yet, under Jewish law, of what is called infanticide or abortion. It is fobidden by Jewish law. The question, however, is whether Jews may not come to certain conclusions with regard to restricting population growth. Such restriction may not be good for the Jewish people, and I am against zero-population growth for the Jewish people; we have had too many losses, and we have to repopulate the earth. But at least we have an open mind with regard to it and may become more liberal with regard to planned parenthood and the circumstances under which abortions may be permitted.

An example of the sociological approach is that when a treaty was signed by the nations of the earth fixing the international dateline, Jews accepted it as part of their Sabbath calculations. If you cross the international dateline on a Friday, for example, you might have lost your Saturday; or, if you came the other way, you might have had two Saturdays in a row. In other words, for Jews, the international dateline became the determining factor for observance of the Sabbath.

The Sabbath is our most cherished and sacred institution. Yet Rabbi Kasher, one of the spiritual giants of Israel, said, "If the day has come when the nations of the earth agree on something—and surely this is a rare phenomenon in itself—we Jews should not be the ones to dissent. Therefore, we should accept it now." That is not a *halakhic* decision. It is purely sociological. We want to support any activity that will bring greater unity among the peoples of the earth. It might very well come to pass that, with regard to certain situations such as abortion, there will be sociological needs that will prompt some compromise in the strictness of the *halakhic* position.

I have alrady touched upon Tay-Sachs disease; but in connection with abortion there are other problems. In addition to the issue of preserving the life of the fetus, is the *quality* of the life to be preserved also a factor? Rabbi Yaakov Emden—although his was a minority view—once permitted a woman to have an abortion in a case where there was no problem with the health of the mother or the child. The problem was that the child was illegitimate, and the mother simply didn't want to raise an illegitimate child in an environment in which the child would suffer ostracism or discrimination. In other words, the potential damage was not physical but psychological.

Today, of course, we regard the physical and the psychological as interconnected. When we speak of the quality of life, we refer to both. If one may perform an abortion to avoid a child who might suffer Tay-Sachs disease, then it may also be proper to abort a fetus that may be psychologically crippled in Jewish society.

The psychological approach has also been used in Jewish law. I urge it in connection with restoring the annulment of marriages. One of the reasons that Jewish law abolished the annulment of marriages was that there was no central court system. It could occur that a rabbi in one part of central Europe would come to one conclusion, and a rabbi in eastern Europe to another. A person who moved from one place to another would find that the annulment was not recognized. (And this is a problem in the United States, where divorces granted in one state are not always recognized by another state.) Realizing that an annulment might not be recognized, the rabbis abolished the entire concept. Today, however, with a central authority in Israel, it is possible to restore it, under the aegis of the Supreme Court of Israel. But this also is based on a psychological factor, one to which Jews are responsive.

An argument advanced by the rabbis in the Talmud for permitting women release from unfortunate marriages was that the woman could have entered the marriage under a mistaken impression. She had thought the man was healthy and now discovered that he was not. That, argued some rabbis, would be enough to invalidate the marriage. The Talmud, however, would not permit such invalidation, on the grounds that a woman prefers any kind of marriage to no marriage. That psychological assumption may have been true 1,000 years ago or possibly 500 years ago. It surely is no longer true. If the psychological assumption is changed, you can change the rule.

We now come to the teleological approach, by which one thinks of the rules as serving certain purposes. The question is: What was the rule's purpose? If it's no longer serving the purpose, or if there's a greater purpose to be served, then we may revise the rule.

There is the story of a man who said that he would die unless he could cohabit with a particular woman. The doctors agreed that this was so. No rabbi would have bothered to consider the case if the judgment had not been rendered by competent physicians that the man's life was in danger. After discussing the case, the rabbi refused to grant the man's request under any circumstances. The doctors suggested that if the woman at least exposed herself, this might save the patient. The rabbi forbade this.

We have to accept the premise that the doctors made a valid medical judgment that the man's life was in danger. Yet the sanctity of his life was ignored. The rabbi said, in effect: We will not permit women to be demeaned and denigrated this way; the daughters of Israel will not be used for this kind of purpose. The rabbi's judgment assigned to the *quality* of life—the quality of women's lives in Jewish society, and the standing that they enjoyed—primacy over the *saving* of a life that, in the opinion of the doctors, was in danger. Here is a veering between antonimies where one value yielded to another.

In an article which I wrote on the subject of violence, I said that in connection with many values, or activities of the human being, we have poles. Judaism never said of anything: This is absolutely forbidden. There are circumstances in which practically all rules are suspended. What we want is the control of basic instincts. Jews, like other human beings, are expected to eat. We suggest, however, that they eat in a Torah way that will lend dignity and sanctity to the process of ingestion. We want men and women to cohabit, and not just for procreation, but for pleasure; but we want them to do so in a way that lends sanctity to the relationship, and not as physical gratification with occasional ensuing disgust. We know that people, by nature, engage in violence; but the violence must be limited to certain circumstances.

This raises the question of suicide. To what extent may men and women engage in violence against themselves? That is a deep *halakhic* problem. There is a classic case in the Talmud which once again indicates the extent to which most issues represent gray areas, rather then black and white. There are two men in a desert; they have enough water for one of them to drink and survive. If both drink, they both will perish.

Ben Petura said, "Let them both die rather than that one shall be responsible for the death of his brother": an heroic point of view. Rabbi Akiva said, "No! There is no moral or ethical obligation for a man to sacrifice his life. He's allowed to drink, even if it means the death of his brother. Because the Torah says, 'Your brother shall live *with you*.' Your life has priority; therefore, you're allowed to drink the water."

The commentators have been nonplussed that Maimonides did not cite this case. Rabbi Moshe Feinstein, a great authority in our century, said that Maimonides didn't have to, because he had already elsewhere stated that a poor man has a prior right to charity. A poor man has to take care of himself first. If survival depends upon water, then he is poor. He has to take care of himself first. Maimonides therefore did not have to repeat the rule in application to two men in the wilderness about to perish because of the lack of water.

Another authority, the Minchat Chinuch, finds Ben Petura's view more interesting: One man shouldn't see the death of the other. But what if one of the two is a child? Shouldn't the adult give the water to the child? The adult is under an obligation not to see the death of his brother, but the child has not yet reached the age of obligation. Therefore, if it's a child, the adult must give the water to the child. Rabbi Akiva says that even in such a case, a man is entitled to take care of himself first.

I was asked to write a paper on what a hospital administrator should do when two patients need the same machine. Jewish literature (Rabbi Yaakov Emden) in the eighteenth and nineteenth century took the position that, based upon one Mishna, there's an order of priorities as to who has the prior right to live. A 'Kohen' comes before a 'Levi,' and a 'Levi' comes before a 'Israel,' an 'Israel' comes before a *mamzer,* and so on. Males come before females, presumably on the basis of the quality of life: the man who has more *mitzvot* to perform is needed by society more than one who doesn't have as many *mitzvot* to perform. Such was the judgment of one rabbi. But there is nothing in the Talmud to support him even though that *mishna* had been studied for 1500 years before Rabbi Emden.

I read the same mishnah, and was happy to discover that Rabbi Feinstein has interpreted it the same way I did; that it has nothing to do with survival, or the prolongation of life. It has to do with who gets fed first by the social services of the community; whose life will be demeaned more if they have to go around begging? In that case, it might be that a male has priority, because it's more demeaning to him to become a beggar than it is for a woman. In the case of captivity, it's vice versa; you ransom the woman first, because she will more likely be abused bodily than the male. It has nothing to do with physical survival. Thus this process is a dynamic one, and what comes into play are all these factors, psychological and teleological as well.

The Bible, the Talmud, Jewish literature, *halakhic* sources, the *halakhic* process, all provide guidelines for individual decision. These help one to see all sides of an issue. However, there must be consultation with others whose character we admire: the doctor, the patient, the family, the hospital administrator, all must play a role in making the decisions in medical ethics. There should also be consultation with rabbis and ethicists.

One should not approach these problems trivially, as if to say, "Well, a woman's fetus is no different from her hair or her nails. She's in charge of what she's going to do with her nails, and it's the same with her fetus." There should be no participation of government in this process. Jewish law provides virtually no penalties, when the issue is purely moral. For a doctor who performs an abortion, there is no punishment in Jewish law even when it is prohibited; even when it is a gross violation of Jewish law, there are no penalties.

There is no punishment for the doctor who decides to detach a machine. But this he should do after consultation. Obviously, a hospital administrator should not take the machine away from a young person who is poor to give it to a donor to the hospital who has just been brought in. If he makes that decision, he ought be called to account by a committee at the hospital. defend himself as to whether he acted in good conscience. It is the conscience of the person who is acting that is the important factor. The state cannot provide guidelines or mandates. The decision is between a man and God.

One might question whether my attitude is an Orthodox position. Is it perhaps closer to the Conservative position? I don't know. I am not concerned with labels. I know that my position is supported by *halakhic* sources. The real difference among rabbis—and I hate using the adjectives Orthodox and Conservative and Reform—is the readiness with which they are prepared to ignore existing principles and values, and simply say: we're living in a modern age; we know better; this is our age and the decisions are altogether ours.

We must remember that, as far as the Jewish tradition is concerned, utilitarianism may play a part; but it is only a part. Above and beyond utilitarian needs and demands there are concepts of holiness. Among these concepts are the sanctity of life, the sanctity of human society, and especially the sanctity and eternity of the Jewish people.

11

The Ethical Implications of New Reproductive Techniques

Rabbi David M. Feldman, D.H.L.

Professor Alex Capron, formerly of Georgetown University and now here at the University of Southern California in a new capacity as professor of Law and Medicine—dealing with the interface between legal and medical implications of continuing developments in the field—used a graphic metaphor to describe where we are. Our response to new problems in medical ethics, he said, is like seeing a taxi parked at the end of the block; you hasten to come closer and get into it; but just as you reach it, it pulls away from you at 90 miles an hour. That's the nature of our subject today. We will focus on some ethical implications of the state of the art, only to watch it get away from us and leave new aspects unresolved.

It has been some years since that historic moment in Oldham, England, when Drs. Steptoe and Edwards announced the birth of the first "test-tube baby," the result of their pioneering efforts at in vitro fertilization. When the achievement was made public, the *New York Daily News* convened a symposium to discuss the theological implications of the process, and I was invited to join with a Protestant and two Catholic spokesmen on the panel. I remember my surprise to hear the Catholic authorities express their opposition to in vitro fertilization, in view of the Church's well-known "pro-life" position. If abortion is to be disallowed in the name of sustaining potential life, I thought that laboratory assistance towards the same end ought to be welcomed. Instead, they opposed it on grounds of violating "natural law;" that life should be sustained only in the natural manner, and any deviation from the natural process of fertilization and gestation is a violation of this theological principle.

I responded that "natural law" may indeed be a philosophic consideration in Catholicism historically, but Judaic morality does not recognize the concept of natural law as a binding principle; on the contrary, we are bidden to overcome nature and natural law. To worship nature is pagan; to be dominated by it is also wrong. The proper teaching is associated with the midrashic application of a verse in Genesis. In the narrative concerning the Creation, the biblical text tells us that God "ceased from all His work, which God had created to do *(asher bara Elokim la'asot)*." What is meant, asks the Midrash, by "created to do"? It means He created the world with much more left "to do"; but, having created Man, the work will be finished by Man. Hence we are "partners with God in completing the Creation," in continuing the work of creation. Nature is not sovereign; it is in the service of man. We are to control nature, not be controlled by it. This is what mandates our use of lightning rods, our damming rivers, even our use of heaters and air conditioners. Circumcision, too, implies that nature or the body need not be taken as is. If blocked Fallopian tubes impede the natural process of fertilization, or if sperm must be strengthened by combining ejaculates, there should be no objection to making use of the laboratory or the Petri dish under these circumstances. This, too, is a matter of controlling nature, especially in view of the desirability of the goal, namely making conception possible.

The point is further illustrated by the example of contraception. Use of the birth control pill was opposed by the Church on grounds that it too violated natural law. Other means are onanistic, but even the pill is unacceptable because it allows a process to begin while making impossible its natural culmination. The natural end result of an act of intercourse is supposed to be at least the possibility of conception; when this is prevented, natural law is violated. (An irreverent response to this objection was voiced by N. St. John Stevas in Britain, who wrote that this means gum-chewing should be forbidden. Since chewing sets in motion the process of salivation, chewing gum sets in motion a process that will never culminate in the expected swallowing and digestion.) Though the oral contraceptive does not constitute a mechanical barrier or impediment, it does make the end result of conception impossible.

By contrast, when the contraceptive diaphragm became available, its use was permitted by Rabbi Mordecai Schwadron on the grounds that violation of the natural process is immaterial. Just as, he argued, marital relations are permitted when one's wife is already pregnant, so are they permitted when her condition is made to resemble that of pregnancy. The mitzvah of *onah,* of ongoing marital relations, is independent of the mitzvah of *p'ru ur'vu,* of procreation; hence onah is permitted and even encouraged during pregnancy. (Marital relations have two coequal purposes: procreational and relational. Especially during pregnancy, when she "loses her figure," the sexual relationship expresses reassuring love.) The diaphragm closes the uteral os; in pregnancy, the uterus is also "closed." There is no difference, argues Rabbi Schwadron, between a natural condition of closed uterus, such as pregnancy, and an artificial one, such as with the use of a diaphragm. The pill causes the reproductive system to simulate a physiological condition of pregnancy; the diaphragm can be said to do so anatomically. The exigencies of the situation allow us to use other-than-natural means to prevent conception, and certainly to make conception possible through in-vitro fertilization.

The in-vitro procedure is then a meritorious deed in that it helps the couple fulfill both its procreative mitzvah and desire. It has in fact been superseded in some quarters by in vivo fertilization, which has the advantage of avoiding surgery, for the fertilized ovum can be lavaged out and implanted in the womb of another. But this technique, as well as related ones of embryonic transfer such as surrogate or host motherhood, raises troubling questions of maternal identity. In the Talmud's imagery, "There are three partners in the birth of the human child,"—the father, the mother, and God. The mother actually gives more. The genetic endowment of the father is matched both by the mother's genetic endowment, the ovum, and by her gestational environment, the womb. If these two contributions are divided between two women, one supplying the ovum and the other the womb, which, now, is the mother? Moreover, in the case of surrogacy, where both of these contributions are offered back to a third party, a sponsoring couple, what maternal claim accrues to the sponsor?

Even these ultramodern phenomena have their precedents in Scripture. Rachel and Leah had their own children but, before and in between these births, they "sponsored" children through their handmaidens Bilhah and Zilpah. These handmaidens, as well as Hagar in Abraham's day, were prototypes of surrogate mothers; and, going beyond the text to Midrashic elaboration, a child of Leah's was conceived in the womb of Rachel, giving us an early case of in vivo fertilization or embryonic transfer. But these instances were free of the sociological problems that complicate the picture today. The "surrogates" did not have a change of heart and insist on keeping the babies, nor did the "sponsors" renege because the babies were not up to their expectations. More important, there was no financial arrangement.

Surrogacy today involves payment of a fee, and the fee is very much part of the problem. It enters the category of baby bartering, which may violate the 13th Amendment against purchase of a human being. On the other hand, the fee may, as in adoption, be for incidental expenses. The American College of Obstetricians and Gynecologists issued a policy statement by its executive committee in May of 1983, in which were listed several hesitations and guidelines concerning surrogacy. We permit our members, it said, to counsel infertile couples who wish to sponsor, or fertile women who wish to accommodate, providing there is no financial exploitation; there should be no fee beyond the expenses for travel, lab tests, etc.; and both parties must agree contractually to all specifics. The "worst-case scenario" that was feared was that either the host mother would renege because she had grown attached to the child, leaving the sponsors bereft, or that the child might be born defective and the sponsoring parents would renege, leaving the host mother with a defective child that was very much hers. What actually happened in America was worse than the "worst case." The host mother gave birth to a severely handicapped child and insisted that the sponsors live up to their agreement and take the child. It was subsequently proven clinically that the child was the offspring of the host mother and her own husband, with whom she had relations during the time of the agreement, in violation of the express terms of that agreement.

For reasons such as these and others, the Warnock Commission of the United Kingdom issued its report in the summer of 1984, in which it recommended against surrogacy altogether. Rabbi Immanuel Jakobovitz, Chief Rabbi there and an authority on Jewish medical ethics, responded enthusiastically. "To use another person as incubator," he said, "and then take from her the child she carried and delivered, for a fee, is a revolting degradation of maternity, and an affront to human dignity." Because of the many and complex legal and moral problems associated with the idea of a surrogate mother, we place this at the bottom of the hierarchy of available options to satisfy a couple's desire for a child.

But embryonic transfer arrangements, when protected from abuse, can be an acceptable solution to problems of conception. The question of maternal identity can be resolved in either direction, based on the following arguments: The sponsoring mother, in whose womb the conceptus is fertilized, can be termed the "natural" mother because the genetic, as opposed to the gestational, contribution is the more dynamic one, supplying the all-important genetic code. Also, the donated zygote can be said to be a nascent being already, with the identity of the child already intact. Further, the first mother's role is not replaceable by technology, while the second mother's is: the gestation could conceivably be done in the laboratory.

On the other hand, maternity can be claimed for the host mother on these grounds: a transplanted organ becomes an integral part of the body of the recipient, which means that the recipient of an ovarian transplant would become the mother. Also, the host mother gives both nurture and gestation to the embryo. As a Congressional committee was told in August, 1984, "the biological fact is that the gestational mother has contributed more of herself to the child than the genetic mother, and therefore has a greater biological investment and interest in it.'' Moreover, the legal presumption in favor of the host mother ''gives the child and society certainty of identification at the time of birth, which is a protection for both mother and child.'' With good arguments on both sides, some Israeli hospitals where in vivo fertilization has taken place, list both mothers on the birth certificate. For the first time in history, while we make our way through the mind-boggling implications of new developments in reproductive technology, babies are recorded as having two mothers. Two maternal relationships, like that of mother and father, may exist simultaneously.

Of course, Jewish law would never sanction recourse to any such methods merely to spare one the inconvenience of pregnancy and childbearing, and certainly not in order to insure some package of genetic characteristics, such as blue eyes or tall stature. But where the natural alternative is not available, these resourceful ways of bringing about the desideratum become acceptable. Enabling a woman to fulfill the maternal yearning, or a couple to fulfill the *mitzvah,* is itself a *mitzvah.* Accordingly, our Medical Ethics Committee has made explicit what is implicit in Jewish legal tradition. We have declared ''barrenness'' to be an ''illness,'' a loss of normal health. The principle whereby all the ritual and other laws of the Torah are set aside to cure pathological conditions, therefore, are likewise to be set aside to overcome infertility.

Before in vitro or in vivo fertilization were a gleam in anyone's eye, assistance to procreation was found in artificial insemination, either of a husband's immotile sperm (AIH) or of a donor's sperm (AID) when the husband was infertile as well as impotent. These procedures bring in tow a different set of halakhic and moral problems, though AIH much less so. Problems with the latter involve mainly the procurement of the semen; that is, the avoidance of onanism. Also, the unwitting or deliberate admixture of the semen of another, to increase fertility strength, is certainly unacceptable. But where the husband's semen alone is procured in a nonmasturbatory way, the insemination itself and the subsequent developments are free of halakhic or other complications.

It is AID that represents a series of problems. Some Rabbinic authorities declare the process adulterous and the offspring illegitimate. Others remind us that adultery is a conscious violation of the marriage vow by illicit intimacy, none of which takes place in this clinical procedure; hence no adultery or illegitimacy can be associated with artificial insemination by donor. Nonetheless, it does sever the human, family bond, and—more serious from the standpoint of practical consequences—it does conceal paternity. When the children grow they may unwittingly marry their siblings, meaning that unknown paternity has led to the grave sin of incest.

Adoption of a born child, then, might seem the better alternative, though the objection of unknown paternity applies here, too. Hence the identity of natural parents should be knowable to the child, or to a readily accessible friend, to avoid the incest contingency. In the opinion of one psychological school of thought, adoption is preferable because it avoids resentment by the husband. If his wife required artificial insemination by another, the child will at least bear her genetic endowment, which is a plus; but it leaves the husband out entirely, which is a minus. Where the child is adopted, neither parent has genetic input, which is a minus; but it eliminates resentment or jealousy, or a constant reminder of the husband's disproportionate inadequacy, which is a plus.

Professor Leon Kass has reminded us of another dimension. It is not only unknown or uncertain paternity or maternity that gives us pause, but the absence of identifiable ancestry. The concept of *yichus* of lineage is not one of elitism, but of taking pride in specific parents and grandparents, and seeking to carry forward the ideals or qualities associated with them. *Yichus* adds to the humanness of reproduction, which is in danger of being lost through these new techniques. But again, where there is no alternative, these represent a distinct gain, on balance, provided they are zealously guarded from abuse.

12

Visiting the Sick
An Authentic
Encounter

Rabbi Levi Meier, Ph.D.

As Chaplain of Cedars-Sinai Medical Center, I take care of
four major areas: religious institutional policy and procedures, religious services, seminars on Jewish medical ethics,
and pastoral visitations. This volume has focused on the
difficult and complex decision-making processes involving
physicians, patients, and family members.

Another major area of medical ethics is the *routine* care
of patients. This requires that the professional give adequate
time to the patient, and see him or her as a *person*. Most
of my time at the medical center is devoted to pastoral visitations in situations of presurgery anxiety, postsurgery
depression, and major illness. In the course of this experience I have developed guidelines formulated to assure that
the visit be of maximum benefit to the patient, and these
are here described.

Within the range of human relationships, the "classical
medical model" and the "authentic engaging encounter"
are at opposite poles of the continuum. The classical medical

model draws a sharp division between the doctor and the patient. The doctor metacommunicates that he knows more about the patient than the patient himself does. Frequently, medical theory and technology take precedence over direct interaction with the patient. This position allows the doctor to evaluate, diagnose, judge, and disclose the patient's illness to the patient. The patient frequently feels helpless in that he must rely on the doctor's expertise (Ofman, 1976).

Contrary to this approach is the "authentic engaging encounter," which can come about between any two people, regardless of their professions or any supposedly hierarchical relationship. In a medical encounter of this type, both the doctor and patient realize that all humans must ultimately face similar life situations. The quality of the relationship between the two is one of reciprocal mutuality—each party declares what he really is all about. The doctor is willing to unmask himself and share with the patient his own fears and trepidations. Within this intimately engaged encounter, the patient realizes that his recovery, or, more specifically, his will to recover, is a responsibility shared by doctor and patient. A common encounter situation that has not been widely dealt with from the point of view of Jewish law is that of visiting the sick. Psychological insights into the *Halakha* (Jewish law) of visiting the sick (Shulhan Arukh, Yoreh Deah, 335), clearly indicate that the relationship between the visitor and the patient ought to be an authentic engaging one.

The laws of visiting the sick emphasize three aspects of this situation: an authentic relationship is the central core of the visit; both the visitor and patient share life's uncertainties and fears, and the visitor must strive for the ability to demonstrate genuine empathy.

The fact that the relationship both prior to and during a person's illness is the basis of and related to the efficacy of the visit is demonstrated by detailing which friends are allowed to visit immediately, and which after a 3-day period (Shulhan Arukh, Yoreh Deah, 335.1).

Those people who have had a prior relationship with the patient can visit immediately. However, those people who are merely acquaintances, who ordinarily see the patient sporadically or incidentally can only visit after the first 3 days of illness. If a relationship exists, it makes sense to continue it during a difficult and trying period. The patient feels comfortable enough to share some of his inner thoughts with such a confidant. However, a period of illness is no time to intensify a relationship with a casual acquaintance. This attempt would probably only make the patient uncomfortable.

In addition to specifying on which days it is permissible to visit, the Halakha also recommends which hours in the day are most suitable for the effectiveness of the visitor-patient relationship. The visitor should not visit during the first 3 or the last 3 hours of the day. During these time periods, the patient will appear, respectively, too well or too sick, and the visitor will not be moved to pray on behalf of the patient either because he looks so healthy, or because he looks so sick that prayers are too late (Shulhan Arukh, Yoreh Deah, 335:4).

During the course of the day, however, the health status of the patient will appear such that the visitor will be emotionally moved to pray on his behalf. Thus, the day and time specifications for visiting the sick reflect a genuine caring relationship between patient and visitor.

The visitor should not conceal his intention to pray on behalf of the patient. The visitor should pray for divine mercy in the language that the patient understands, despite the fact that prayers are generally recited in Hebrew. When the patient hears and understands what is being requested on his behalf, his feelings of isolation and of being forsaken are alleviated.

The reciprocal relationship between visitor and patient is so crucial that the visitor must consider on which occasions it is inappropriate to visit the sick. Any visit that would possibly cause embarrassment or impose other hardship is forbidden (Shulhan Arukh, Yoreh Deah, 335:8).

For example, visiting one who has an intestinal disease that might cause him embarrassment, or one who suffers from headaches making speech difficult should be avoided. A visitor is not just paying a visit to an object, but to a subject—a person with a specific condition and unique feelings.

The halakha's concern about the I-Thou relationship (Buber, 1970) between patient and visitor is not limited to the here and now, wherein one person is sick and one is healthy. The vicissitudes of life dictate that one day the visitor will be the patient and the patient will be the visitor. Our common human frailties are at once recognized by both visitor and patient in an authentic encounter.

Throughout "healthy life," unspoken differences are usually noted between people of different socioeconomic status (SES), as reflected in peer socialization. In contrast to this approach to social behavior are the halakhic guidelines for visiting the sick. Since man is finite, all aspects of SES vanish in the face of illness. A person of prestige is obligated to visit a youngster, and all other human differences are set aside during a person's health crisis (Shulhan Arukh, Yoreh Deah, 335:2).

We are all vulnerable to illness. A powerful person may tomorrow be in the throes of death. Illness is the equalizer of all human beings. Since we are all in the same boat, genuine empathy for the pain and suffering of the patient must be felt and understood.

In the course of a visit to the sick, clichés and trite statements are usually inappropriate and change the relationship from an I-Thou to an I-It encounter. It makes no sense to quote theological truths to a person in agony. The Midrash relates:

> Rabbi Hanina once fell ill. Rabbi Yohanan went to visit him. He said: "How do you feel?" Rabbi Hanina replied: "How grievous are my sufferings!" Rabbi Yohanan said: "But surely the reward for them is also great!" Rabbi Hanina said: "I want neither them nor their reward!" (Song of Songs, Rabbah 2:16:2).

Yes, the reward for suffering is great (Talmud, Brachos 5A). But this Talmudic opinion, which Rabbi Hanina obviously knew, was meaningless at that time. A dictum that is appropriate in a classroom may be totally inappropriate for consoling a person in anguish. A suffering person desires to be understood. His pain, his anger with God, his blasphemies, must not be challenged but must be accepted at this time. An illustration of this situation is given in the Midrash:

> Rabbi Simeon ben Yohai used to visit the sick. He once met a man who was swollen and afflicted with intestinal disease, uttering blasphemies against God. Said Rabbi Simeon: "Worthless one! Pray rather for mercy for yourself." Said the patient, "May God remove these sufferings from me and place them on you . . ." (Abot de Rabbi Nathan 4:1).

A sick person desires the visitor to be able to demonstrate genuineness, warmth, and empathy (Truax & Carkhuff, 1967). Again, it is these qualities that create an I-Thou rather than an I-It relationship.

How should the visitor feel about himself after he has accomplished his task? Lest he feel grandiose and view himself as the provider of health, the halakah dictates that he feel humble and recognize the efficacy of the only Healer—God. This end is served by regulating where the visitor may sit. He should not sit higher than the sick person, because the Shekhinah is above the head of the sick (Shulhan Arukh, Yoreh Deah, 335:3); that is, the restoration of health is dependent upon God.

The halakha recognizes that no human relationship can ever be dictated. What can be *suggested* are guidelines making possible human relationships of an I-Thou nature. Most discussions of this precept detail three responsibilities involved in visiting the sick: performing personal tasks for the patient; encouraging the patient; and praying for his or her recovery (Rosner, 1977). These acts, however, are merely outward manifestations of the precept. Behind them lies the "essence" (Van der Leeuw, 1963) which has been described. If the visit is performed in bad faith (Sartre, 1967), it is antithetical to its purpose. The visitor is challenged to open himself up—to recognize his own deficiencies and weaknesses.

Visiting the sick requires one to recognize and share our common fears, as well as to empathize, and be authentic. In contrast, when one is in the presence of mourners, the only response is total silence and, before departing, the recital: "May the Omnipresent comfort you amongst the other mourners of Zion and Jerusalem " (Ha-Siddur).

Visiting the sick is a difficult commandment to perform. It is among those acts the fruit of which man eats in this world while the principal remains for him for the world to come (Talmud, Shabbos, 127b). It requires an authentic and genuine response between the visitor and patient. The concrete guidelines that the halakha sets before us offer us a way to realize this authentic encounter, the essential component of the visitor-patient relationship.

REFERENCES

Abot de Rabbi Nathan. Standard Edition.

Buber, M. *I and thou.* (W. Kaufman, Ed. and trans.). New York: Charles Scribner's Sons, 1970.

Ha-Siddur Ha-Shalem. (P. Birnbaum, trans.). New York: Hebrew Publishing Company, 1949.

Ofman, W.V. *Affirmation and reality.* Los Angeles: Western Psychological Services, 1976.

Rosner, F. *Medicine in the Bible and the Talmud.* The Library of Jewish Law and Ethics, Volume V, (N. Lamm, Ed.). New York: KTAV Publishing House, Inc. Yeshiva University Press, 1977.

Talmud. Standard Editions

Truax, C.B. & Carkhuff, R.R., *Toward effective counseling and psychotherapy: Training and practice.* Chicago: Aldine Publishing Company, 1967.

Van der Leeuw, G. *Religion in essence and manifestation.* New York: Harper & Row, 1963.

Selected English Bibliography on Jewish Medical Ethics

Abraham, S.A. *Medical halachah for everyone*. New York: Feldheim Publishers, 1980.

Bleich, J.D. *Contemporary halakhic problems*. The Library of Jewish Law and Ethics, Volumes IV and X, (N. Lamm, Ed.). New York: KTAV Publishing House, Inc., Yeshiva University Press, 1977 and 1983.

Bleich, J.D. *Judaism and healing: Halakhic perspectives*. New York: KTAV Publishing House, Inc., Yeshiva University Press, 1981.

Feldman, D.M. *Marital relations, birth control and abortion in Jewish law*. New York: Shocken Books, 1974.

Feldman, D.M. & Rosner, F. (Eds.). *Compendium on medical ethics* (6th edition). Federation of Jewish Philanthropies of New York, 1984.

Gribetz, D. & Tendler, M.D. (Eds.). Medical ethics: The Jewish point of view. *The Mount Sinai Journal of Medicine,* January-February 1984, *51*(1).

Jakobovits, I. *Jewish medical ethics: A comparative and historical study of the Jewish religion attitude to medicine and its practice*. New York: Bloch Publishing Company, 1975.

Preuss, J. *Biblical and Talmudic medicine*. (F. Rosner, trans.). New York: Sanhedrin Press, Hebrew Publishing Company, 1978.

Rosner, F. *Modern medicine and Jewish law*. Yeshiva University Department of Special Publications, 1972.

Rosner, F. *Medicine in the Bible and the Talmud*. The Library of Jewish Law and Ethics, Volume V, (N. Lamm, Ed.). New York: KTAV Publishing House, Inc., Yeshiva University Press, 1977.

Rosner, F. *Medicine in Mishneh Torah of Maimonides*. New York: KTAV Publishing House, Inc., Yeshiva University Press, 1984.

Rosner, F. & Bleich, J.D. (Eds.). *Jewish bioethics*. New York: Sanhedrin Press, Hebrew Publishing Company, 1979.

Rosner, F. & Tendler, M.D. *Practical medical Halacha*. New York: Rephael Society, Association of Orthodox Jewish Scientists, Feldheim Publishers, 1980.

Rothkoff, A. Visiting the sick. *Encyclopedia Judaica*. Jerusalem: Keter Publishing House, 1972.

Soloveitchik, J.B. The lonely man of faith. *Tradition*. 1975, 7(2)

Waldenberg, E.Y. On death and dying. In *A concise response: Jewish medical law*. (A. Steinberg, Ed., D. Simons, trans.). California: Gefen Publishing, 1980.

Index*

* Names of authors cited in footnotes, references, or bibliography are not listed.